To Dad, because we care —

Happy Birthday!

Love,

Helen + John

eat,
drink,
be merry,
and
live longer

eat,
drink,
be merry,
and
live longer

Harry J. Johnson, M.D.

DOUBLEDAY & COMPANY, INC., GARDEN CITY, NEW YORK

Foreword

Eat, Drink, Be Merry, and Live Longer

Do you fear old age? Many people do. Some have seen loved ones deteriorate with multiple afflictions, "alive but not living." Others have seen associates "suddenly" fail shortly after retirement and not enjoy the fruits of their labors. Medicare has brought the plight of many of our old people to our attention so graphically that some people say, "I don't want to live out my years. I'd rather die young."

These are natural, understandable reactions. But they represent a confusion between chronological old age and senility. Senility can strike early or it may not strike at all.

To me, the fact that many old people don't get adequate medical attention is only part of the problem. What worries me is how so many of them got into such poor health that they require so much medical assistance.

Statistically, the number of years each of us is likely to live is pretty well established. What is not established is the proportion of years that will be spent in vital living and those spent nursing infirmities of old age.

The big news is that so-called old age need not happen to you. You have a good chance to stay middle-aged for life.

I say middle-aged—not young. We cannot recapture youth, but there are now ways to stretch out and prolong those wonderful middle years throughout the balance of your life. And I think that this is what most of us want, once we have tasted the enjoyment, the appreciation, and understanding of life that comes in the years after forty.

As an article in *Time* expressed it, "One of the philosophical satisfactions of middle age is not being young. The sign of emotional health for the middle-ager is that he prefers his own age; he has no desire to go back to twenty because he knows what twenty is in a way that twenty does not. It is difference in perspective: youth's is flat, middle age's is three-dimensional. It is the difference between ignorance and wisdom, impulse and judgment. The young think there is no tomorrow; middle age knows there is tomorrow and tomorrow and tomorrow. The young want to dynamite the treasure vaults of life; middle age has learned the combination. The young think they know; middle age knows that no one knows."

Middle age is when most people are at the height of their powers, when life, though sometimes hectic, is most exciting. One feels the excitement of accomplishment and the feeling that he is climbing higher and higher. It is akin to a mountain ascent. Sometimes the path is steep, sometimes it's a gentle rise, but the movement is upward. Anxious as we are to get to the summit, we always wonder, will we find a plateau or an abyss? The plateau is middle age, the abyss is senility. But, unlike the mountain climber, you can control which it will be.

Again, using the mountain climbing analogy, there are many perils along the way. Unless you are well equipped and knowledgeable, you will not survive the climb. It is in middle age that we encounter the biggest roadblocks to health. This is when the degenerative diseases attack—coronary heart disease and cancer—the two biggest killers in modern America.

Yet, you can get around these roadblocks and you can stretch out these pleasant and productive years far beyond anything ever dreamed of by man. The way has been prepared to virtually eliminate "old age" as we have known it through history.

If we can achieve this, think what it can mean. It would be a double gift. The individual could look forward to an extension of life free from the worries of incapacity and the worries of how he will care for himself. And in his own middle years he would be relieved of the burden of taking care of the elderly ahead of him.

The fear of old age hangs heavy over mid-century America. Fortunately, its elimination is within our grasp.

The power to achieve middle age for life is here now. It is not a drug, it is not an electronic device, it has nothing to do with computers or special foods. It is not complicated and it is virtually free of charge.

It is, simply, a distillation of medical knowledge that has been accumulated over the years.

There is only one person is the world who can put this knowledge to work for you.

You are that person.

This is a bold assertion. But if you will review with me the advances that have been made in medicine, you will see how I arrive at this.

In the twentieth century more advances in medicine have been made than in all the centuries before. One result is that a child born in America today has a life expectancy of about seventy years. In 1900 it was only forty-nine years.

The twentieth century has seen the development of penicillin, sulfa drugs, insulin, and undreamed of surgical techniques. As a result of millions of dollars spent on medical research, the public now finds "wonder" drugs commonplace.

Popular articles and lectures lead many people to believe that modern medicine can heal or repair almost any human ailment.

This, of course, is not true—even though the curative powers of modern medicine are indeed remarkable. Yet curative medicine is not alone responsible for the fantastic gains in life expectancy. These have been won largely through advances in *preventive* medicine, and the heroes were laboratory researchers, the so-called "microbe hunters."

We must remember that at the turn of the century the killers were outside agents which attacked the body. Their main victims were infants and children. The researchers first went to work to discover the bacteria and viruses causing these diseases. Then they developed vaccines which would prevent the occurrence of the diseases in the first place. Today's children, through immunization, can be protected from diptheria, smallpox, polio, and most of the other diseases which attack from outside. Most of the deaths which still occur from these diseases are due to failure to use the preventive measures which are ready and available.

Another group of people who have contributed to our present state of health and long life are in the public health field. Only when we have a cranberry scare, or a sudden outbreak of food poisoning at a picnic, do we appreciate the protection given us by public health inspectors in our food stores and (other) restaurants. Typhoid was largely eliminated by the imposition of sanitary measures and the development of pure water supplies. Such public health measures are of a preventive, rather than a curative, nature.

It is clear, then, that our sensational rise in life expectancy stems both from preventive and curative medicine. Vaccines, immunizations, improved sanitation, informative articles regarding healthful living habits, all of these are, in a sense, preventive measures.

With all of the progress in preventing and treating disease the millennium in medicine is not yet here. For some born with a predisposition to diseases such as diabetes and high blood pressure unavoidable infirmities may appear during later years. Cancer has eluded the most scrutinizing research. Arteriosclerosis, arthritis, alcoholism respond poorly if at all to therapy and preventive measures have not been very effective.

As each decade passes more people will live into the eighth decade but with the added years will go added health problems. Deterioration is inevitable but the rate is, to a degree, within our control.

We now have improved means for diagnosing diseases and disorders early enough to permit successful treatment. One hundred years ago it would have been meaningless to have diagnosed a brain tumor because no one knew what to do about it. So it is the preventive medicine approach, backed up by the application of medical knowledge and surgical skills after diagnosis, which has brought us to our unparalleled standard of health and longevity.

What has happened, then, is that we have learned to prolong life—increase the life expectancy for everyone far beyond what we have dreamed to be possible. But in so doing, we have neglected the *quality* of life. It is not enough to keep a person living, we must make the living worth while.

Once a person has accumulated the multiple ailments we now associate with old age, it is too late. It is much like an automobile. We have all seen a two-year-old car that has been neglected and abused sent to the junk heap. Yet there are Model T Fords still running as well as the day they were built. With cars, we call it preventive maintenance; with humans, preventive medicine. The principle is the same, but there is one essential difference in the analogy.

A car cannot maintain itself. It requires mechanics.

But doctors are not mechanics for humans. True, they can do marvelous things when a person is ill or has an accident. But they cannot replace parts and make you good as new. Nor can they keep you in good running condition. Only you have that power.

The purpose of this book, then, is to share with you the essential information you need to remain middle-aged for life. One word of caution: The *simplicity* of the rules of health may startle you.

If you are looking for some "magic"—some dramatic and offbeat approaches—this book is not for you. All you will find are the basic rules to which almost all competent medical authorities will subscribe.

Can anyone use these rules? Yes. Of course, the younger you are, the more effective they will be. A man in his sixties can still buy life insurance, but the premiums are prohibitive. He benefits most if he starts young—at least by thirty-five. The same is true in health. The time to prepare for middle age for life is before you've reached the middle years.

The root structure for infirmity with advancing age is set decades earlier. It is our aim to prevent these roots from being established and, if already present, to weed them out before they can prematurely choke off the productive potential of middle age.

But, regardless of your age, if you are in reasonably good shape now, the recommendations in this book will help you to prolong your well-being. And that is the "secret" of staying middle-aged for life.

Contents

Contents   xiii

Eat, Drink, Be Merry, and Live Longer

*This is one of the oldest bits of health advice
in recorded history. In only seven words,
it links together the basic physical needs
of mankind. It is the heart of this opening section
which reviews the "rules" of health.*

1. Eating

Eating Should Be Fun

Of the making of diets, there seems no end. If primitive man, who ate when he was hungry—and whatever was available—could see us now, he would wonder why so much fuss about such an instinctive matter as eating.

There appears to be a diet to fit every person in the country—to take care of every whim, indulge every desire for faddism.

It's about time that we recognize that there is nothing inconsistent between good nutrition and the enjoyment of eating, just as long as you let the bathroom scale be your guide as to what and how much you eat.

Strictly speaking, "diets" are for sick people, children, pregnant women, and for persons for whom proper nutrition poses a problem. The great preponderance of the one hundred million adults in this country are normal healthy people. This country of ours has the most fantastic array and abundance of food in the world.

It is an insult, if not fraudulent, to be told that we need to follow special "diets" for good health.

Generally speaking, these special diets make one of two assertions.

1. That certain foods are so important that they must be eaten to the exclusion of other foods.

2. That a certain combination of foods will provide a painless, effortless way to better health.

Both assertions are completely false.

No one food is nutritionally so superior that it belongs on every person's table. Yes, oranges are high in Vitamin C, but so are parsley and peppers. So the chances are that if you enjoy eating and eat what you enjoy you will assimilate all of the nutrients necessary for good health.

Malnutrition is not only a matter of undernutrition, it is more often a matter of overnutrition. Here the affluent are worse off than the poor. Overnutrition, the product of overeating, produces overweight, shortens life, contributes to degenerative diseases such as high blood pressure and diabetes and indirectly to coronary heart disease, the Number One killer in the United States.

As to weight control, this is a serious problem, as we will discuss later, but here too the answer is not a "magic" diet. Rather, it is simply eating more of the lower caloric foods, less of the fats, and drinking less alcohol. In recent years, people have recognized the high caloric content of alcoholic beverages. Naturally, they are attracted to a diet which promises them weight control by continuing their normal consumption of alcohol and cutting down on carbohydrates. But, this so-called "drinking man's diet" is simply another way of cutting the total caloric intake.

It is often said by nutrition experts that the answer to better health lies in variety of food. This brings to the minds of most of us the thought of "balanced" meals—a certain amount of vegetables, fruits, eggs, meats, etc., each day. This is good, and housewives know that variety makes the preparation of the family meal more interesting.

Some Basics of Nutrition

There are six main food components: carbohydrates, fats, proteins, vitamins, minerals, and water. Practically every food contains several or all of these groups in varying amounts.

Carbohydrates, fat, and protein contribute calories (fuel of energy and the wherewithal for growth and replacement of worn out tissues). Carbohydrate foods (sugar and starches) are the most plentiful source of energy, usually furnishing 40 to 50 per cent of our caloric intake. See the complete table of the calorie, carbohydrate, fat, and protein content of common foods in the Appendix, at the end of this book.

Fats are more concentrated sources of calories, yielding about twice as many calories as do the same amounts by weight of either carbohydrate or protein. On a weighted basis, fat sources in the diet may yield several times as many calories as carbohydrate or protein foods because the last two contain appreciable amounts of water that "dilute" the caloric content. However, in typical American meals, fats provide 40 to 45 per cent of our calories. The balance of our calories, 10 to 15 per cent, comes from protein.

If the weight is above normal, the most efficient way to bring down the level is by curtailment of the fat intake. Nutritionists are urging that the fat intake should be reduced to about 30 to 35 per cent of our total calories.

There is an easy way of achieving proper nutrition. Nature has been so bountiful that the vital nutritional elements exist in a great many different foods. Thus even a person with limited food interests—the so-called "meat and potatoes man"—can achieve adequate nourishment and still follow his taste desires.

Let us not forget that eating is instinctive and natural. Many people try too hard to achieve a balanced diet and end up disliking eating. But, if you simply let your taste be your guide, and eat enough of the foods you enjoy, the chances are good that you will be well nourished.

No One Way to Good Nutrition

Admittedly, some people, through bad examples, develop poor eating habits and may thus lack proper nutrition. Also there are food faddists who insist that certain foods are superior to other foods which contain exactly the same nutrients.

A young college girl came to see me one day because she was twenty pounds above her best weight and was anxious to get back to normal. In discussing her eating routine she stated that she ate only the "healthiest" kinds of food, and that was why she was overweight.

Since I was very interested to learn about the "healthiest" kinds of food, I asked her to tell me about them. She first stressed the value of whole-wheat bread and volunteered the information that white bread was not worth eating, "because all the nutritional value has been refined out of it." She also prided herself upon using only "natural" sweeteners, such as honey and maple syrup, and she again volunteered that "white sugar was not fit to eat."

There were many other very positive opinions offered with regard to the virtues of some articles of food and condemnation of others. It was a little shocking to me to hear so much misinformation from a person so young. Yet it is not surprising when we consider some of the information broadcast on radio and television by self-styled nutrition experts. A warped conception of what constitutes good nutrition is the too frequent result. For many years white bread and white sugar have been condemned by these so-called food experts.

From the time man began to cook his food bread has been outstanding in its position as the staff of life. Today there is a tendency to de-emphasize the importance of bread as an essential part of the day's food intake because of enthusiasm for weight reduction. Nutritionally and calorically it is hard to beat bread as an article of diet.

All bread is nutritionally good and can fit into any dietary routine whether for weight gain or weight loss or weight maintenance. It makes little difference whether it is whole-wheat bread, rye, or enriched white bread. A slice of each has essentially the same proteins and the same over-all nutritional value. And let me emphasize again, enriched white bread is just as nutritious as any other type of bread.

All of the common types of bread are equally well digested, but the white bread made from enriched, refined flour has some advantages over the others. It is usually better tolerated by those who have difficulty with their digestion. Toasting does not alter the nutritional value or the digestibility of bread.

White sugar is pure carbohydrate food, the most inexpensive energy producer that we can get. It is a natural food, the product of sugar cane or sugar beets. It is not manufactured, as has been popularly believed. Those of us who are a little overweight have to be a bit cautious in the indulgence of sugar. Nevertheless a dessert now and then or a piece of candy is food for all of us, and what would desserts be like without sugar? Everything we eat does not have to be loaded with vitamins and minerals to be considered worthy of the name food. When you want a sweetener there is none better than plain, pure white sugar.

Food Fads Can Be Dangerous

Not long ago my newspaper contained this headline: "Cult Diet Studied in Jersey Death—Woman, 24, Believed to Have Died of Malnutrition."

The story related how for nine months this young woman had been following an all-cereal regimen as part of a "macrobiotic" diet developed by a Japanese. The medical examiner observed that her weight had declined markedly from her normal of 130 pounds. While he had not completed his formal report, his preliminary diagnosis was "acute starvation."

The misguided victim found her diet in a book which describes "macrobiotic medicine" as the "art of rejuvenation and longevity." The book offered dietary remedies for a number of illnesses ranging from apoplexy to varicose veins. It condemned such foods as cow's milk, sugar, red meat, and a number of vegetables, including potatoes, tomatoes, and eggplant.

This is but the latest tragic incident in the history of food faddism. Typically, the faddist extols the exceptional nutritional values of some types of food and promotes and promises cures of disease by diet. Actually, the only diseases cured by diet are the deficiency diseases caused by improper or inadequate eating. Remember, the primary interest of those promoting food fads is to sell a book or a product. Your health or well-being is not of their concern.

Some years ago we had the blackstrap molasses and wheat germ fad foisted on the public. More recently we had the vinegar and honey nonsense promoted with an air of authority. There is no food that has any special health value, nor any drink that has any special health benefit. All clean food is health food. Special grinding or mechanical mixing processes do not improve the nutritional value of food. The only thing that is special about these touted preparations is the price.

Developing Good Eating Habits

More people have gotten off the track because some well-meaning person kept preaching "eat it because it's good for you." The normal person, if left alone and presented with a choice of a variety of food, will select through taste what's good for him. The easy natural way to achieve normal nutrition through eating is to let your taste be your guide. Keep in mind that I am talking about the "average" person who has no weight problem. I once knew a man who preferred his soup at the end, instead of the beginning, of the meal. Admittedly this is eccentric, but it made absolutely no difference to his nutritional needs.

Neither am I talking about taste in a gourmet sense. If you have developed a highly sophisticated taste for food, you will perhaps enjoy eating more than most people. And that is all to the good. However, keep in mind that the stomach cannot differentiate between a filet mignon and the cheapest chuck roast. There is plenty of nourishing food in this world for every taste and pocketbook.

How Important Is a "Good" Breakfast?

A "good" breakfast is an old American custom and represents a meal of substantial caloric value. It dates back to colonial times when the working day was long and labor was arduous. Huge amounts of food, six thousand calories or more, were necessary to satisfy a person who worked twelve to fourteen hours a day.

The tradition of the "good" breakfast was based upon a need for lots of food and not any special benefit of a large meal at the beginning of the day. The penalty of large meals when accompanied by the easier, more affluent life became evident during the first quarter of this century. Life insurance companies noted an increased mortality among the obese and the country became weight conscious.

Our dining habits today are dominated by the pleasure of eating, not by the need to provide energy for work. A word of caution, however. Our appetites and desires are not fully dependable guides to our nutritional needs. Health examinations of executives indicates that 70 per cent are overweight, 30 per cent markedly so. A logical step to control overweight is to limit the amount of food at meals that are least interesting and least enjoyable.

Surveys show that more than half the adult population in America eats a light breakfast. Based on studies of executive health, I find that those who regularly limit breakfast to a piece of toast, fruit juice, and coffee are as healthy, vigorous and free from disease as those who eat more. There is no health benefit, then, to be gained by eating a "good" breakfast.

There are many reasons why people prefer a light breakfast. A desire to control weight is most frequently noted, and nothing could be more commendable. Sometimes the appetite for breakfast is so poor that the pleasure of eating is limited. Occasionally, the time for eating is short so that the scanty intake simply takes less time.

We recommend, then, that you let your weight and your eating time preferences determine what foods to eat and when. The body can adapt to almost any routine of eating hours and food distribution. Aside from the discomfort of hunger pains, it does no harm to skip a meal now and then, or to set aside a day for a very low ration.

The Pleasures of Eating

The enjoyment of food is not merely a taste sensation. It is a blending together of three different senses, each one alerting the other—the scent of food, the sight of food, and the taste of food. To a lesser degree hearing and touch come into the consciousness of eating, too. We all can recall the inviting sound of the sizzling steak and the softness of the light soufflé. The degree to which each of the senses enters into the act of eating determines the total satisfaction and pleasure of the meal. All should be satisfied, none should be satiated. Whenever the senses are delicately teased, the pleasure of anticipation is intensified and the joy of participation is increased.

Some people look upon eating as a refueling operation. They

approach the table as they would a gasoline filling station. The only objective is to "fill 'er up." There are also people who resent the time devoted to eating. Some, I believe, would welcome a magic pill to provide the essentials for energy and growth, so that the time given to eating could be saved. Fortunately, no such magic pill will ever be created. There is no better expenditure of time than that devoted to leisurely partaking of the greatest blessing conferred on man—food.

There should be a nice balance between anticipation of food, actual eating, and the delightful satisfaction and contentment that follow. For some, anticipation provides the greatest pleasure. The mere thought of good food is exciting fun. For others, this pleasure is provided in the actual eating. And, for still others, it comes from the pleasant satiated sensation that follows.

We must realize, of course, that everything we do for pleasure, if abused, will result in displeasure. The glutton suffers the unpleasant aftermath of overindulgence. The chronic overeater accumulates fat and weight and thereby shortens his life expectancy and sacrifices many of the comforts and other pleasures of life. There is a direct correlation between the amount that is eaten and the pleasure that is derived. Maximum pleasure always comes from moderate intake. Eat until the appetite is satisfied, never until it is nonexistent. There is much to be said in favor of the philosophy of "live to eat," even though it has been criticized frequently. How absurd! As if the joy of eating is something to be considered indecent or unworthy! We feel sorry for those who eat merely to live.

And I'd like to add a word of praise for the china, glassware and silver industries which emphasize the importance of an attractive décor in the dining room. The pleasant atmosphere which they aim to achieve acts for the enjoyment of a meal and good digestion afterward. Add cheerful, optimistic companions and the picture is complete. One "sour" person in the group can ruin the fun for all and cause indigestion for most. The long face should be relegated to the solitary refueling department.

Conclusions

•There is nothing mysterious about good nutrition. It simply comes from taking advantage of all of the wonderful foods which this great country of ours makes available.

•No food furnishes all of the nutrients required by the body.

•If there are some foods you honestly do not like, don't feel guilty. There are many others which will meet your needs.

•Avoid the food faddist who proclaims that a certain concoction is necessary to good health. Spurn the fanatic who offers food supplements and additives. The normal person does not need to add anything to his food.

•Forget about "health" foods. All clean food is health food.

•The average person should forget about "diets." Diets are for abnormal conditions. The normal person should concentrate on eating for pleasure.

•Malnutrition includes overnutrition as well as undernutrition. And more of us are in danger of overnutrition. Therefore, consult the bathroom scales regularly.

•A variety of foods consumed will give you a proper balance in the needed carbohydrates, fats, proteins, minerals, vitamins. But don't make a fetish of trying to get an exact balance.

•Eat for enjoyment and enjoy what you eat. Let your taste guide you to the foods you need for good nutrition.

•There's a most popular cookbook called *The Joy of Cooking*. Actually, for the objective it is trying to reach, it might be titled *The Joy of Eating*. Either way, approaching cooking and eating with a sense of pleasure, makes for The Joy of Living.

2. Do You Need
Vitamins?

It is a ludicrous situation when the citizens of the best-fed nation in history dose themselves with food supplements such as vitamins. Fortunately the practice is not harmful except to the pocketbook, but it is certainly unnecessary. One reason for the habit may be that vitamin users do not understand what vitamins really are.

Perhaps the purpose of vitamins will be clearer if we review the circumstances under which one important vitamin—B1—was discovered. We choose this example as a tribute to Dr. Robert R. Williams, the American scientist who died recently. When he was only twenty-four, he was a fledgling scientist in the Orient. Appalled by the death toll from beriberi, he tried an experiment of his own with a Filipino baby dying of the dread disease. He forced a few drops of brown rice bran (the husk coating of the rice) down the throat of the gasping infant. The symptoms cleared within hours.

For the next two decades Dr. Williams worked to find the special substance in the bran which conquered the killing disease. The special "something" turned out to be thiamine chloride, which we now know as Vitamin B1. It is present in brown rice, but not in the milled and polished rice which the world's billion rice eaters eat. Subsequent experiments by Dr. Williams in the Philippines showed that the polished rice could be enriched by the addition of Vitamin B1, restoring what was lost by milling.

The same principle is now used by American food manufacturers so that much of the bread and other foodstuffs we consume have been enriched with Vitamin B1 and other vitamins. It should appear obvious, then, that, since so many of our foods contain vitamins naturally and others are enriched, there is no need to buy vitamins by the bottle. Let us review, then, the basic points which Dr. Williams' findings revealed.

First, vitamins are naturally present in foods and they are natural and vital ingredients to proper nutrition. The average person who eats a variety of the foods which nature offers will obtain more than enough vitamins. The Irish, for instance, are not blessed by oranges, but they have never suffered for a lack of Vitamin C because Vitamin C is also present in cabbage. It is only when a diet is severely restricted, such as that of the Oriental rice eaters—and the particular foodstuff is deficient in vitamins— that food should be supplemented with added vitamins.

The American food industry has been very alert to new developments in nutrition. The result is that it is difficult to buy food in America which is not rich in vitamins, either natural or added, as in bread, milk, and cereals. And if you will read the fine print on some food labels, you will note that the exact vitamin content is described along with a notation about the daily vitamin needs of most people. It is clear that the vitamins supplied are more than ample.

Why Are Vitamins So Popular?

Why, then, do people insist upon consuming additional vitamins by the bottle? There are several reasons. Some of my patients tell me that they believe vitamins relieve "sluggishness" and fatigue.

There is no foundation in fact for this. Others believe that vitamins prevent colds. Again there is not the slightest bit of evidence to support this contention. But the man who has been taking vitamins and has been fortunate enough to avoid a cold during the winter will be a vitamin consumer for life.

People are more health conscious than they used to be and they have more money to spend on themselves. Vitamin manufacturers naturally do a lot of persuasive advertising and, since their products are harmless, they are perfectly within their rights. But the beneficial effects of supplemental vitamins on the health are grossly exaggerated in the minds of many people and often are purely coincidental—like the man who sprayed his apartment against elephants and sure enough, he was never bothered by elephants.

But surely, you may ask, there must be some use for vitamins. Of course, but only in abnormal situations. If the person has a restricted diet, or in childhood, or in the senior years when some people are careless about eating the right foods, or in pregnancy, or following certain illnesses—all these are times when supplementary vitamins are useful and necessary and sometimes lifesaving. But these are all special situations where the physician should make the decision as to the amount and the kinds of vitamins required. Self-dosing with vitamins is not justified.

Conclusion

•Put another way, the use of vitamins by healthy people who enjoy their meals is primarily of psychological benefit. It is an unnecessary habit and can be costly. Fortunately, vitamins are eliminated rapidly, and an overdose won't hurt you. So if every winter your wife insists that you start taking vitamins, don't argue, take them. You may not be healthier, but your life will be more harmonious.

3. Overeating: America's Number One Health Hazard

Eating should be fun, but in abundant America overeating has reached epidemic proportions, creating our Number One health hazard. More than half the people in the world are suffering from undernutrition. Yet one in four Americans is a victim of overnutrition, a disease that is just as devastating.

It is a chronic disease, one that will stay with you for life, and hasten your death, if you let it go untreated.

It is a maimer that can rob you of your attractiveness, a crippler that can rob you of your effectiveness, a killer that can rob you of your life.

We spend more than a half billion dollars per year combating its symptoms the wrong way. Yet the disease itself can be cured—permanently—not only without cost but actually with measurable dollar savings.

Overnutrition is a nutritional disease that stems from abundance just as rickets, scurvy, and yaws stem from deprivation. Overnutrition is habitual overeating, taking in more calories through food and drink than the body needs or can put to good use.

The word "habitual" is an important part of the definition because overnutrition is a chronic rather than an acute disease. The sudden bulge that results from an eating and drinking spree can be reduced just as quickly with emergency measures. But the bulge that appears with middle age or even earlier, and increases slowly but surely with the months and years, cannot be cured with diets or pills or steam baths.

Since overnutrition results from eating too much, the cure is simple and logical: learn to EAT LESS, not as a crash, emergency measure but permanently, habitually. As Dr. Frederick Stare, the Harvard nutritionist, puts it, overweight results not from what you eat and drink between Christmas and New Year's, but from what you eat and drink between New Year's and Christmas.

I have proposed to hundreds of patients that they learn to eat less. Often they react like this:

"But, Doctor, is it worth it? I enjoy eating and drinking. It helps me relax, to overcome the tensions of my job . . ."

I assure them that a sensible eating pattern is far from a starvation diet. It can be a thoroughly enjoyable three meals a day, with even that relaxing end-of-the-workday drink. As to the importance of weight control, I suggest that they consider these facts:

Not only does overweight interfere with fitness and attractiveness, but there is a definite correlation between overweight and shortened life expectancy. For each 10 per cent increase above normal weight, the mortality rate increases 20 per cent. Heart disease, kidney disease, strokes, and diabetes occur two and a half times as frequently among persons 25 per cent over normal weight than among those of the same age whose weight is normal. In fact, overweight is directly and indirectly responsible for more disability and illness than any other disease. It has been correctly called the Number One health hazard of our time.

And then I point out to them that, the sooner the cure is started, the easier it will be to carry out. Sensible eating can become a habit, just like overeating, and the resultant feeling of fitness can be much more rewarding than the temporary pleasures of lemon meringue.

Sometimes they say, "This is fine for a lot of people, but not for me. Weight runs in my family. It's inevitable. It would be a waste of time for me to try to reduce."

I have to tell them, simply and bluntly, that this is poppycock. Congenital overweight is nothing more or less than a congenitally good appetite unharnessed by will power.

Or they may attribute excess weight to a glandular condition. In well over 95 per cent, thorough examination reveals a perfectly normal glandular system that is working overtime in a futile attempt to prevent accumulation of unnecessary pounds under a constant barrage of excess calories.

Now what about you? Are you suffering from O-N (over-nutrition)? The later stages are obvious, not only to you but to the world. The early stage, however, may be noticeable only to your tailor or dressmaker. As the ads used to put it, even your best friend won't tell you. And yet, as in the case of many chronic diseases, the earlier O-N is detected, the easier it is to cure.

You don't need a doctor to detect O-N in its early stages. All you need is a bathroom scale and a weight chart. Weigh yourself once a week (on the same day of the week and same time of the day) and enter your weight on the chart presented here. Now you have taken the guesswork out of detecting O-N. Here is what your chart will tell you.

First Degree O-N

If you are five pounds above your normal weight (as determined roughly by the table or, more accurately, by your doctor), you are suffering from FIRST DEGREE O-N.

Consider the added five pounds as a warning that many more will follow unless you adopt and maintain this simple cure:

Cut out all between-meals snacks. Eat three meals a day—generous portions but no seconds.

Get into the habit of a balanced diet. You don't have to consult food charts to achieve this, nor do you have to supplement your diet with vitamins. Just make sure that your daily diet includes something from each of these groups: meat, fish, or eggs; milk or cheese; fresh fruits; green and starchy vegetables; whole-grain cereals. There is no need to eliminate any type of food (even bread, potatoes, or sugar) or to concentrate on certain so-called "health foods." Balance your diet and eat in moderation—and you can eat what you like.

If your weight chart shows a drop of even a pound a month, you have successfully caught O-N in its early, easily curable stage. Maintain this new eating habit for life and you may have no more weight problems.

Second Degree O-N
(up to 25 per cent above normal weight)

But if you don't make this relatively easy adjustment in eating habits soon enough or conscientiously enough, the figures on your weekly weight chart will continue to climb. You will have to face up to SECOND DEGREE O-N and the need for a more strenuous change in your way of eating and drinking.

Your goal now should be gradual but steady weight reduction—a pound a week or five pounds a month. A crash diet, pills, or any other emergency measure at this point would be silly; stop the measure and the pounds would come rolling back. Weight must come off as gradually as it was gained, if it is to stay off.

Now, to lose weight safely and sensibly, learn to remove fat from meat, to make butter or margarine a rarity and dessert a treat reserved for very special occasions. Eat vegetables in smaller portions, and not creamed. The calorie chart will tell you that potatoes, peas, and corn must give way to green leafy vegetables,

WEEKLY PROGRESS CHART

WEIGHT AT START_____ GOAL_____

WEEK	WEIGHT	WEEK	WEIGHT
1ST		27TH	
2ND		28TH	
3RD		29TH	
4TH		30TH	
5TH		31ST	
6TH		32ND	
7TH		33RD	
8TH		34TH	
9TH		35TH	
10TH		36TH	
11TH		37TH	
12TH		38TH	
13TH		39TH	
14TH		40TH	
15TH		41ST	
16TH		42ND	
17TH		43RD	
18TH		44TH	
19TH		45TH	
20TH		46TH	
21ST		47TH	
22ND		48TH	
23RD		49TH	
24TH		50TH	
25TH		51ST	
26TH		52ND	

WEIGHT TABLE

TABLES FOR HEIGHT AND WEIGHT
WITHOUT CLOTHING

MEN					WOMEN			
Ft.	In.	20 yr.	25 yr.	30 yr.	Ft.	In.	20 yr.	25 yr.	30 yr.
		98	102	105			90	92	95
5	0	108	113	117	4	8	100	103	105
		122	127	131			111	116	119
		100	104	107			91	94	97
5	1	111	115	119	4	9	102	105	107
		124	129	133			113	118	121
		103	106	109			93	96	99
5	2	114	118	122	4	10	104	106	109
		128	132	137			117	121	123
		105	109	112			95	98	100
5	3	117	122	124	4	11	105	108	111
		131	137	140			119	122	125
		108	113	116			98	99	102
5	4.	121	125	128	5	0	108	110	113
		136	141	144			122	124	127
		112	117·	119			100	102	105
5	5	124	129	132	5	1	111	113	116
		140	145	148			125	127	130
		116	120	123			103	105	109
5	6	128	133	136	5	2	114	117	119
		144	149	153			128	131	134
		119	124	125			105	107	110
5	7	132	137	140	5	3	117	120	123
		148	154	157			131	135	138
		123	126	129			107	110	113
5	8	136	141	143	5	4	120	123	125
		153	158	162			135	138	142
		125	130	134			111	114	117
5	9	140	144	148	5	5	124	126	129
		157	162	166			139	142	145
		127	134	138			115	117	120
5	10	143	149	153	5	6	127	130	133
		162	167	172			143	146	150
		134	139	143			118	121	124
5	11	148	154	159	5	7	131	134	137
		166	173	179			147	150	154
		138	143	148			121	124	126
6	0	153	160	164	5	8	134	138	141
		172	180	184			151	155	159
		143	149	153			124	127	129
6	1	158	165	170	5	9	138	142	143
		177	185	191			155	159	162
		146	153	159			127	130.	133
6	2	162	170	176	5	10	142	144	147
		182	191	198			160	162	165
		151	158	163			132	133	136
6	3	167	175	181	5	11	146	148	151
		188·	197	204			164	167	170

1 - Light Frame   2 - Medium Frame   3 - Heavy Frame

and apples and oranges should replace bananas and grapes. One highball with water is perfectly permissible if it helps you relax at the end of the day, but hold it at one and forget sweetened cocktails—and no cheese and crackers with the drink.

Third Degree O-N
(more than 25 per cent above normal weight)

These relatively easy adjustments in your caloric intake should enable you to combat O-N successfully. But if your weight has climbed to 25 per cent above normal, face up to the fact that you are suffering from Third Degree O-N—a real and serious health hazard that may require treatment under a physician's direction. He may prescribe diet or medication or both. Whatever he prescribes, be prepared to follow his orders to the letter; they could save your life.

Can you face up to overnutrition as a chronic disease and change your habits, permanently, to overcome it?

Only you can answer this question.

If you are like most people, you will first try to ignore the existence of your weight problem, and then seek some easy way around it.

I am sure you know the portly executive who takes his little bottle of sugar substitute from his pocket, dutifully drops a pill into his after-lunch coffee—and proceeds to enjoy his parfait. Others look to the steam bath, the swimming pool, the golf course as substitutes for sensible eating and drinking. Invariably these crutches serve to salve the conscience of the overeater but do nothing for his weight problem.

Moderate exercise is an important step toward over-all fitness. But attempted weight reduction through exercise alone is ineffective. Chances are you will quickly take back in liquids the weight you lose through perspiration. And unaccustomed strenuous physical activity can put an additional burden on a heart already over-worked by O-N.

Similarly, massage and steam baths can help achieve muscle tone and a feeling of fitness. But the workout will not materially affect weight, nor will gadgets that claim to jiggle, bounce, or pound you into slimness.

The single best exercise in a weight-reducing program is walking an hour each day. It has been estimated that this will result in a pound loss every month. Not much, you say? Over a year's time it equals twelve pounds, a twelve-pound loss over and above the product of your calorie reduction routine.

Should You Count Calories?

While it's calories we're talking about, to keep track of each day's intake serves no useful purpose. A rigidly planned diet with counted calories will accomplish a loss of weight, but it will also remove the pleasure from eating. This kind of dieting dignifiies the whole concept of weight reduction far beyond the point it warrants. A simple and effective routine is changed into one which creates a sense of virtue in the dieter and a virtue of this kind usually has a short life. During the dieting period the convert sometimes becomes a bore—he talks and destroys not only his own eating pleasures but those of his fellow diners as well.

What about Special Diets?

As for "crash" or "elimination" diets, you can expect to gain back any weight you lose as soon as you stop the diet. Meanwhile, you are probably depriving your body of proteins, minerals, or vitamins that are necessary to a balanced diet.

The "drinking man's diet" is a case in point. It is just another in the procession of fad diets that promise a painless, quick way to lose weight. Any recommended routine that condones the misdeeds of its followers will inevitably be popular. But, like all its predecessors, it is doomed to an early demise. To condone the excessive consumption of alcoholic beverages indicated in sample menus of this diet is courting serious trouble. You may wind up becoming an alcoholic.

The menus of the "drinking man's diet" provide approximately three thousand calories per day, about one-third of which is contributed by alcohol. It is unlikely that one can lose much weight in such a regimen.

This diet unrealistically recommends that its followers restrict their intake of carbohydrates to sixty grams per day. If adhered to for more than a short time, this regimen could result in nutritional deficiency. Whiskey is no substitute for carbohydrate.

Alcohol calories are merely unwanted fellow travelers. They are also "empty" calories, containing neither minerals nor vitamins. Consequently, to include alcoholic calories in a reducing routine is more objectional than to include calories from ice cream or potatoes. It makes no sense to cut down on good and necessary carbohydrate food in order to allow for excessive indulgence in alcoholic beverages.

Also stay away from reducing pills that can be bought without prescription. They are usually worthless. Any effective reducing medicine is too dangerous to be taken without the direction and close supervision of a physician. I have heard of people using reducing pills that have been prescribed for friends or relatives, without even undergoing a doctor's examination themselves. I can think of few more dangerous practices. Self-medication is always dangerous. It can cover up symptoms that would warn the physician of a potentially serious organic disease. It may lead you to habit, leaving you in worse shape than ever when the support collapses. And there is always the risk of side effects, for only the physician, with your personal medical picture in mind, can determine what it is safe for you to take and what the dosage should be. Only a thorough physical examination and knowledge of your medical history as well as your working, living, and eating habits can enable the physician to prescribe a safe and effective reducing program for you.

Recognize your weight problem for what it is—a treatable chronic condition. Approach it with will power and good sense and you will add many full and enjoyable days to your life.

Some people wonder if it's necessary to be under the care of a weight-reducing specialist in order to lose weight. The answer is emphatically no. It is neither necessary nor desirable.

The doctor who specializes in weight reduction engages in a rather dubious specialty that commands little respect from his medical colleagues. The doctor is merely a benevolent policeman to whom the overweight victim reports for gentle discipline when results are not up to the expected. When progress is satisfactory, of course, the doctor is profuse in his compliments. In either case, his charges can be substantial.

To be sure, there are a few situations when a physician's help is necessary. When obesity is a manifestation of glandular dysfunction, the attention of an endocrinologist is essential. And when obesity is related to emotional illness, a psychiatrist can be very helpful.

But the overwhelming majority of overweight people do not need the services of an endocrinologist, psychiatrist, or weight-reduction specialist. The doctor adds no element of safety to their own efforts to lose weight.

One final word. When you have lost ten or more pounds and your friends come forward with compliments, accept them graciously and gratefully. But resist the overpowering temptation to describe in detail just how you have accomplished this momentous feat. Your objective in shedding weight should be the improvement of your health and life expectancy, not to provide a topic for conversation with which to bore your friends.

Conclusions

• One in four Americans is a victim of overnutrition—a serious disease which will hasten your death.

• If you are as little as five pounds overweight, you have taken the first step toward obesity. And if you are 25 per cent above normal weight, you are in serious trouble and need the immediate help of a physician.

4. Drinking

Alcohol has been used by man since the beginning of time, but not always wisely. Learning how to drink is one of the keys to a healthier and happier life.

How to Drink and Stay Healthy

Have you ever thought of anything as pleasant as drinking leading to a disease that is incurable? This, unfortunately, is the truth about alcoholism.

Let it be clear at the outset that this is not a Prohibition treatise. But, if you yourself drink at all—and if members of your family use alcohol—you ought to know the medical facts about alcohol.

Despite all efforts to identify and treat alcoholism, the number of victims is increasing. What is worse, the chances are poor that many of them will be cured or even deterred by present means of treatment.

Let us remember, however, that the spectacular increase in life expectancy during the first half of this century did not result from successful treatment of disease. Present longevity was made possible through preventing disease. Since prevention has been so effective in other diseases, it is high time we made an all out effort to prevent alcoholism.

One of the tricky aspects in discussing alcoholism is getting agreement on the cause. Certain research authorities tell us that alcoholism is a disease and that alcoholics are sick people. They consider the cause to be, not alcohol, but certain qualities or defects in the emotional or physical make up of the victim. To be sure, there are factors such as tolerance to alcohol, vicissitudes of life and emotional stability that contribute to alcoholism. Nevertheless, without the consumption of alcohol, there can't be alcoholism. One must drink alcohol to become an alcoholic. Hence any program of alcoholism prevention must make its primary target the control of alcohol consumption. We say control, not prohibition. Alcohol, along with food, fire, and water, is part of man's life. Used properly, they all contribute to life and its enjoyment. Uncontrolled, they will destroy.

The first fact we must recognize is that alcoholism is never acquired innocently and it does not appear spontaneously. It requires great perseverance at heavy drinking to establish the addiction. With very few exceptions, every alcoholic is personally responsible for his alcoholism.

What Is Alcoholism?

What is this disease called alcoholism? What happens to the body when addiction takes place? Addiction is an accommodation by the body to the presence of a drug. Addiction is believed to be brought about by an insidious change in cell metabolism. The cells of the human body are adaptable and can accommodate to a changing environment such as that brought about by alteration in the constituents of the blood. When alcoholic beverages are consumed at frequent intervals, a significant concentration of alcohol is maintained in the circulating blood. The cells of the body accommodate to this new constituent and addiction to alcohol may be established. At this stage, elimination of alcoholic beverages becomes extremely difficult, if not impossible.

In simpler terms, when alcoholic beverages are consumed to such a degree as to interfere with normal home life, business activities, or a person's health, the disease—alcoholism—is present.

Are some people alcohol prone? Psychiatrists tell us that a specific alcoholism-prone personality cannot be identified. We can, however, pinpoint the group from which all alcoholics originate: the heavy drinkers. All alcoholics are heavy drinkers, even though the great majority of heavy drinkers are not yet alcoholics.

It is generally believed that alcoholics are people who have been unable to cope with problems and responsibilities and therefore drink excessively to escape. To be sure, there is a group of young, immature people who learn early that alcohol can isolate and insulate them from the world they live in. Alcohol provides such persons with a readily available means of escape from problems. This, then, is self-medication by a mentally sick person who is in need of psychiatric treatment.

But the great majority of alcoholics are middle-aged people who have been well adjusted and successful with no problems to run from. They have gradually slipped into a way of life that lends itself to heavy drinking. After some years a significant number of them become alcoholics. This is the group with which we are primarily concerned.

Why People Drink Excessively

Why do people drink excessively? Because alcohol is readily available and they like to drink. Alcohol creates an aura of contentment and a release from awareness of responsibilities. A few drinks encourage sociability and help provide a congenial atmosphere. Most people accept this as an experience that is pleasant but temporary. However, when a person seeks to capture and maintain this pleasant state of unreality by continuous drinking the danger of alcoholism is great.

Since alcoholism is a direct consequence of excessive drinking, the incidence of alcoholism will parallel that of heavy drinking. The intelligent indulgence in alcoholic beverages never results in alcoholism.

Recognizing First Signs of Alcoholism

The danger arises when the moderate intelligent drinker increases his consumption of alcohol. A personality metamorphosis begins to take place. There is an insidious, almost imperceptible change in his pattern of life. A person who once had multiple absorbing interests gradually changes to one in whom alcohol dominates all pleasure and relaxation. He soon looks rather disdainfully upon his more conservative friends and refers to them disparagingly as "two-drink" people. He no longer has time or interest for golf or concerts or the theater. More and more of his leisure time is devoted to drinking until it finally becomes his single-minded interest.

Social Customs and Alcoholism

Why has there been such an increase in the number of heavy drinkers? One reason is that alcoholic beverages are more and more identified with leisure time. Golf has its nineteenth hole. Refreshments after tennis, swimming, and other sports are usually alcoholic beverages. Alcohol is often the constant companion of the card player and the TV watcher. Unfortunately, just plain sitting and drinking has become sufficient unto itself as a leisure time occupation. Even though whiskey is expensive, this is not a deterrent. Economic affluence contributes to alcoholism.

Along with leisure time there is boredom, and alcoholic beverages have become a favorite antidote. Leisure time, affluence, and boredom, then, are probably the primary factors contributing to excessive drinking.

In my opinion, however, the greatest stimulus given to excessive drinking is social acceptance. If we really want to help the heavy drinker to modify his intake we must stop condoning his misconduct when intoxicated. He should not be granted complete immunity from responsibility for his acts. When we speak with amusement of the heavy drinker as "tight" or "high," we dignify a very undignified state. Actually the heavy drinker, when intoxicated, assumes the role of the alcoholic, not a very attractive part to play. At best heavy drinkers are horrible bores and should be made to see themselves in this unflattering condition.

Changing social customs have forced many people to drink who would not do so otherwise. In some "smart" areas of the country, it is incredible to the host that anyone would prefer a nonalcoholic drink. The result is that some people are embarrassed to request a soft drink.

There is much to be said in favor of the old English custom of tea in the afternoon. The caloric value of the tea and the cake is far less than two drinks and actually would be preferred by many people. However, the fear of being considered unsophisticated discourages the hostess and guest alike. This reversion back to an older day may be considered reactionary, but I'm sure many people would be happier.

An intoxicated state does not spontaneously descend upon a person. The effects of alcohol make themselves evident long before intoxication takes over. Getting drunk is a deliberate act. Heavy drinkers are being propelled toward alcoholism by their overhospitable friends who encourage repetition of excesses by urging another drink.

When a person feels pressured into having a drink at lunch and he really does not want it, I have suggested that he tell the host or guest that alcohol disagrees with him. He would love to have a drink, but . . . Or, order a long drink and just sip on it slowly and leave most of it.

Control of alcoholism by various treatments and by Alcoholics Anonymous has not been very successful. The alcoholic himself must sincerely desire to be helped. Most alcoholics do not want to stop drinking. Consequently, help is impossible. When an alcoholic really wants to overcome the addiction, then AA offers an effective means.

What is excessive indulgence? This, of course, varies with the tolerance of the person. Everyone should set as a limit to his drinking that which experience has taught is safe for him, and stop short of this.

In order to determine more accurately what should be considered excessive drinking, we carried out a poll among executives. This was very enlightening. It appeared that excessive drinking was always several drinks more than the polled executive personally consumed each day. The upper limit for a "heavy drinker" was a bottle a day and the lowest estimate was six ounces. We have arbitrarily selected the lowest estimate as our concept of heavy drinking. Anyone who consumes six ounces or more of whiskey a day should consider himself a heavy drinker and therefore a potential alcoholic.

Is This Your Pattern?

It might be well to set down a few guidelines which indicate approaching alcoholism for heavy drinkers:

—If two or three years ago a half hour before dinner was set aside to have a drink, and now this has stretched to two hours and four drinks.

—If two or three years ago dinner was anticipated with pleasure and now there is little interest in food and sometimes dinner is completely omitted.

—If two or three years ago cocktails at lunch were for business entertaining only, and now one or two are routine.

—If two or three years ago weekend consumption was little more than that of weekdays, but now drinking is started in the morning and continues more or less all day.

—If this has been your experience, alcoholism is imminent, if not already present.

How to Tell Whether You Are an Alcoholic

Every heavy drinker should take a therapeutic test to determine whether or not he is an alcoholic. In order to be of value, the heavy drinker must be convinced that such a test is necessary and important.

The test is simple. It merely requires that the heavy drinker declare a semiannual alcohol holiday of not less than one week. If this can be done without unpleasant withdrawal symptoms, without a feeling of martyrdom, and with no obsessive desire to return to drinking when the test period is over, alcoholism is not yet present. For those who have a weight problem—and 60 per cent of executives do—the test provides an added dividend. The thousand-calorie reduction in intake could bring about a half-pound loss of weight each day.

When the time for the test period arrives—and if the drinker then rationalizes and justifies a postponement for any reason whatsoever—he is entering the twilight zone of alcoholism and the point of no return may be near.

Alcoholism is 100 per cent preventable. Heavy drinkers should be mindful of the signs that are evident during the preaddictive phase. At any time during this preaddiction period alcoholism can be prevented by limiting alcohol intake.

While alcoholism is the most serious complication of heavy drinking, other hazards emphasize the importance of a more moderate intake. Many serious head injuries occur when the intoxicated person falls against fixtures in the crowded confines of a bathroom. More and more in physical examinations we are amazed to note the frequency of healed broken ribs detected by routine chest X-ray. And we are all aware that much of the slaughter on the highways is due to intoxicated drivers.

It is noteworthy that people do not realize how many drinks they consume each day. We ask this question of each person examined. Many truthfully say they don't know. I recall one man in particular who reported to me that he began to count the number of drinks he consumed each day, and he was amazed. He stopped drinking immediately and stayed on the wagon for a month. Every heavy drinker would also be amazed at the number of drinks he consumed each day.

Be sure you really want the drink you take. Don't be too sociable or accommodating to your drinking friends. An alcoholic never says "no" to another drink. Do you?

Are Six Drinks a Day All Right if I Never Show the Effects?

Definitely not. Give any excuse you want: you don't get hangovers; your work doesn't suffer; your stomach never acts up; your friends all tell you that you hold your liquor well.

It makes no difference. This excessive daily intake of alcohol can do you serious physical harm in the long run, and I advise you to reduce your intake accordingly.

Excessive drinking can damage your liver. Today, doctors view cirrhosis of the liver as a deficiency disease, with malnutrition as a predisposing if not primary cause. Many heavy drinkers often neglect their diets.

But no well-nourished heavy drinker should thereby take comfort, thinking he can avoid cirrhosis simply because he eats adequately. Any steady and heavy drinker is a candidate for the disease in its less obvious forms. Cirrhosis is a chronic liver disease characterized by an increased amount of fibrous tissue that spreads throughout the liver and impairs its function. A tremendous volume of blood returning to the heart from the stomach and intestinal tract must flow through the liver. This fibrous tissue dams the free flow of this blood, inevitably causing a dilatation of the veins in the stomach and esophagus. Although previously in apparent good health, heavy drinkers in middle age occasionally hemorrhage spontaneously (and seriously) from the lining of their stomachs or from ruptured varicose veins in the esophagus.

Just because you have consumed six to eight drinks a day for many years, have felt quite well, have lost no time from your office, and have not been accused of being tight—this does not mean that the alcohol you have consumed is innocuous. No one is immune to the slowly progressive, destructive effects of long-continued excessive drinking. DEATH RATES FROM ALCOHOL ARE ON THE RISE

According to the Metropolitan Life Insurance Co., the reported death rate from alcoholic disorders has risen steadily in recent years—from 5.5 per 100,000 population in 1950 to 8.7 in 1964, an increase of nearly 60 per cent over the period.

Higher death rates from cirrhosis of the liver with alcoholism accounted for most of the increase, while mortality from the other disorders showed little change during the past fifteen years.

Alcoholics are subject to distinctly higher than average death rates. A recent insurance study indicated that persons with a history of alcoholism experienced mortality two and a half to three times higher than standard risks. The heaviest excess mortality was due to diseases of the digestive system, suicide, motor vehicle accidents, other accidents, and homicides.

A Word about the Lunchtime Martini

For some time I have been asking executives: "Why the martini at lunch?" The answer is always the same: "I entertain so much and it is expected by my guests." Most say they really don't want the cocktail but have it because "the other fellow wants it." An advertising executive said in horror, "Imagine taking a client for lunch and not offering him a cocktail—a shocking thought!" The client's reaction, "I know my host wants a drink, so I have one with him—he's paying for it."

Now how about those who lunch alone, or with a friend, and go "Dutch" on the meal? Many of the men consider the drink as routine as the cup of coffee. Some few of the more immature in mind, if not in years, feel that they "need a couple of martinis to keep going the rest of the day." What a confession of incompetence!

Unfortunately the noontime cocktail on working days is not limited to the middle-aged and older executives who are entertaining customers. Men and women in their twenties and thirties have succumbed, and the younger the victim of this routine the greater the hazard to career and to health.

I'll agree that an alcoholic drink adds a touch of festivity to any occasion, and to omit this gesture might appear inhospitable. It may also be interpreted as a little "cheap" on the part of the host. But this apparently innocuous little pastime can be dangerous and very costly. Intelligent drinking has a place in a well-rounded life, but drinking at lunchtime cannot be considered intelligent. The best to be said for cocktails at lunch is that they can be justified under some circumstances and the risk involved is a calculated one.

How to Drink Intelligently

There are those who contend that the disease of alcoholism begins with the first drink, and actually to suggest a drink is to invite disaster. This I cannot subscribe to. I have never heard of anyone becoming a problem drinker because he regularly had a drink before dinner.

Intelligent drinking involves both when as well as how much to drink. The time to drink is at the end of the business day—not at lunch or after dinner.

The predinner drink should never be rushed. Adequate time should be devoted to allow the drinker to settle into a relaxed mood in an atmosphere of peace and quiet. This makes cocktail time the pleasant experience that it is. A drink or two regularly, even three or four on occasion, provides a pleasant release and makes life a little more cheery.

If your annual health checkup shows no organic disorder, this kind of intelligent drinking will not be a health hazard.

What if You Suspect Your Wife or Husband Is Alcoholic?

Since alcoholism is a disease, you have an obligation to your husband or wife or employees to take preventive steps if you suspect one of them is becoming alcohol dependent. However, the last thing you should do is confront the person with your suspicion. It builds up resentment, and it does no good.

The ideal procedure is to alert the family or company doctor. If the person is having a health examination, call the doctor a few days in advance and tell him the details. If this is not possible, perhaps the minister of your church can help.

Conclusions

•Alcoholism is a serious, crippling disease. It is now in the epidemic stage in the United States. Ten per cent of the population—nineteen million people—are alcohol dependent, and 5 per cent—nine and a half million people—are alcoholic, according to Dr. William B. Terhune, medical director of the Silver Hill Foundation. Dr. Terhune, who has studied and treated 1500 alcoholic patients, confirms our statement that there is no cure. Prevention offers the only hope.

• Alcohol itself is the prime ingredient in the making of an alcoholic.
• Alcohol dependency—drinking on all possible occasions to relieve fatigue or stress—leads to alcoholism.
• Social customs which force alcohol on people contribute to the increase in alcoholism.
• On the other hand, alcohol has a place in the life of every healthy person. Intelligent drinking never hurt anyone and makes life more pleasant.
• The rules of intelligent drinking are simple. If you want to drink and avoid alcoholism, here is all you have to remember:
• Restrict daily drinking to one or two, preferably long, drinks at the end of the day. All other alcohol consumption should be selective, not routine.
• A lunchtime cocktail should be reserved for business reasons only, or on infrequent special occasions—never when alone! After-dinner drinks also should be saved for special occasions only.
• A drink or two regularly, even three or four on occasion, adds to the fun of living. The three and four pose no threat of alcoholism, but there is the immediate hazard of accidents and indiscretions.
• Count your drinks and limit their number to your tolerance.
• If you lose count, stop. You are already beyond your safe limit. Alcoholics never count their drinks.
• Don't "sneak" drinks in the kitchen. Alcoholics always do!
• Don't stop for a "quickie" on the way to the train. Wait until you get home.
• Never order doubles.
• "Never on Sunday" would be a good rule to follow, especially after a "Saturday night!"

5. Being Merry

The injunction to eat, drink, and be merry appears several times in the Bible. In biblical times, there was much less to be "merry" with. Pleasures were simple and work was primitive. Today, with all of our complex ways of making a living and our infinite possibilities for entertainment, millions of people no longer have the capacity to be "merry." Many of these people are tense and jittery. Others are dragging at the heels, always tired no matter how little they do. Many can't sleep at night. And, to a sizable number, the so-called increase in leisure time has provided only worry and unhappiness.

Over-all, the result is a series of health problems that were unknown a couple of generations ago. If you are one of those who are "living it up more and enjoying it less," these next chapters may help you.

How to Live with Tension and Enjoy It

The stereotype of the business executive—in fact the way many foreigners think of most Americans—is of a person under constant tension. He swallows tranquilizers by the bushel, and he drinks gallons of black coffee as he sits late at night at his desk, working himself to death. And to watch certain TV commercials, it seems evident that the entire population suffers from the jitters, raw nerves, headaches, indigestion, and complete inability to sleep.

It is certainly true that many of the people who seek medical advice these days have complaints that can be attributed to excessive tension.

At the same time, working hours are much shorter than they were—coffee breaks are an established routine, vacations are longer and more frequent—and we are constantly reminded that we have more leisure than ever before.

Why, then, do we hear so much about tension and pressure? Part of it is the age in which we live. Instantaneous communication has brought the complexities of the world into every home. Constant crises, transmitted to us in solemn voices and big black headlines, provide an atmosphere of anxiety. Because we experience only the present, the perils of today seem worse than anything that has come before. Yet, as we review the advance of the human race, we have never been more secure.

Without at the moment trying to reconcile these seemingly contradictory facts, let us recognize that people who suffer from symptoms caused by tension are faced with a very real and very disturbing condition. Excession tension can bring about physical ailments, such as indigestion, headache, pain in almost any part of the body, and for people under constant tension, life can be a torture.

However, what is a tension-producing situation for one person, is taken in stride by another. Everyone should learn whether his threshold for tension is high or low.

Stress and Tension—Similar but Not the Same

The human body has been designed to resist an infinite number of changes and attacks brought about by its environment. The secret of good health lies in successful adjustment to changing stresses on the body.

STRESS is the rate of wear and tear on the body. In simplest terms, whatever you do that seems strenuous or wearing is stress. Going out into the cold or the heat produces stress. There is stress on the body from disease, physical or mental effort, crossing the street, or being exposed to a draft. Any emotion, any activity causes stress.

The feelings of being tired, jittery, or ill are subjective symptoms of stress. It is how we react to stress that makes the difference between pleasant healthful living and suffering from a variety of unpleasant symptoms.

Again, stress represents a direct physical attack on the body, and excessive tension is one such stress-producing agent.

What, then, is TENSION? First of all, tension is normal and beneficial. It is part of the normal functioning body—in fact, we cannot live healthfully without it. Tension has been defined as "psychic energy that needs to be released." Tension is that inner drive which is usually considered the mark of a successful person, whether he is a top athlete, a bishop, a business leader, a general. Tension is what makes people "go."

By contrast, many psychotics, such as schizophrenics, experience no tension whatsoever. They live in another world, in almost complete tranquillity.

For some reason, there seems to be a popular notion that tension is bad. This isn't so. Like so many other things in life, tension is only harmful in large doses. A watch spring, for example, cannot perform its function without being under constant tension, but we all know the results of overwinding the watch. It is the same with the human body. Tension that keeps us interested and alert is good and necessary. When we move over the fine borderline where we become apprehensive and anxious and fearful, only then is it bad.

Tension, then, like seasoning in food, gives zest and effectiveness to life. Life without tension is like soup without salt. When we participate in sports or watch a football game, we all become tense.

Under circumstances such as the football game, people aren't conscious of being tense. They only realize it when the grip of tension loosens and they experience a feeling of relief.

Doubtless you can recall many situations when you have been tense and then began to unwind. Perhaps you drove the last hour of a long trip through heavy traffic, then checked into a comfortable hotel room. Gradually you realized that you no longer had to be on the alert and you felt contented and relaxed. These are the good moments of living. But imagine if instead you just couldn't unwind, you couldn't relax even in the comfort of your room, and you lay awake reliving the perils of your trip. This is EXCESSIVE TENSION.

The serious thing about excessive tension is that it can bring about very real changes in the body itself if it persists over a period of time. That is why it is essential, if you have any of the symptoms of excessive tension, to find the causes of the tension as quickly as possible.

The Symptoms of Excessive Tension

The physical symptoms of excessive tension include headaches, fatigue, irritability, indigestion, back pains, insomnia, muscular rigidity.

Any one of these symptoms can, of course, arise from an organic disorder or a disease. But this can be determined by a physical examination. This is why the annual health audit it so important.

We also know that many of these symptoms can arise from an emotional disorder. This is a complicated situation involving a person's entire pattern of emotional stability. It is not as likely a cause as many people seem to think. Excessive tension is more likely to be the culprit.

Our experience at the Life Extension Institute in examining nearly three million persons since 1914 has confirmed that the most common single symptom of excessive tension is fatigue. A feeling of exhaustion may be present during the entire day, yet the person has difficulty in sleeping at night.

Another common symptom is a feeling of chronic restlessness and inability to concentrate. I recall one executive in a large company who told me, "No matter how hard I work, I can't seem to get anything done. I hurry through the day at top speed, but I accomplish little." The layman has a phrase for this: "wheel spinning."

Then there is the so-called tension headache, which people describe as a tightness and pulling and aching in the back of the neck and head. Tension is probably the commonest cause of headache among businessmen. It develops regularly late in the day, but X-ray and examination will not reveal any organic cause.

There are also many characteristic symptoms from the gastrointestinal tract—"indigestion," gas, constipation, and lower abdominal cramps—which may be caused by tension.

Finally, palpitation of the heart accompanied by a sensation of tightness in the chest around the heart area can be the result of tension.

Every one of these symptoms is unpleasant, to say the least. They are also a warning that you may be headed for serious trouble.

While excessive tension can disturb people in all walks of life, we think of it most commonly as an "executive disease." It is fashionable to refer to "the rat race" as the villain, and the ulcer is supposedly the Madison Avenue badge of honor.

How Widespread Is Excessive Tension?

To find out how widespread tension really is among executives
we made a study of six thousand businessmen. Our purpose was to
determine the prevalence and degrees of tension as well as the effects
of kinds of jobs upon tension. The results, which were widely publicized, were gratifying: excessive tension among executives is not
nearly as prevalent as is commonly supposed.

For instance, 78 per cent of the businessmen reported that they
were not working too hard.

Eighty-one per cent said that they liked their jobs very much.

Only 1 per cent reported serious personality conflicts with their
business associates.

The great majority reported good health habits as to sleep,
recreation, eating, drinking, and smoking.

What it boiled down to was this: only 13 per cent of the
executives complained of excessive tension, that they worked under
constant tension.

This was most encouraging and corrected an important misunderstanding about executive life. However, 13 per cent of all executives in the country is still a sizable number of persons to be suffering
from excessive tension. We should do our best to understand the
cause of this excessive tension to reduce the number of sufferers.
The effect on the economy, to say nothing of the human misery
among a family of a tension-ridden executive, is such that we
should make every effort to eradicate tension diseases.

Some Tension Case Histories

Several cases come immediately to mind. I recall John Jones,
an extremely successful executive with a large corporation. John is
what is known as a "hard-running" executive. He has an inner

drive that has propelled him to the top and that makes him impatient for results.

This is an example of the good effects of tension. However, when John came to us for an annual physical, he complained of painful headaches, trouble in sleeping, and increasing irritability with his associates and with his family. It didn't take long to determine that John was now a victim of excessive tension. And it didn't take long either to find out the cause, once we had talked over his usual business day.

John had recently taken over a new division of his company which had a poor profit picture. Even though he worked long and hard, he couldn't seem to make a dent in all of the multiple problems involved. He began to think he was the only person "carrying the load." As his tension built up, he increased the pressure on his staff with resulting ill will and loss of co-operation.

Gnawing away at him also was a fear that his superiors were not happy with his progress. His president was a type who was sparing in his praise and John didn't know where he stood. We suggested to John that he settle this matter immediately with his superiors, even if it meant getting another job.

In a week John came in to see me and already he was beginning to be like his old self. His confrontation with his president had revealed that the company's officers were more than happy with what he was accomplishing, in fact, thought it was "miraculous." The president was so fearful, in fact, that John might leave that he insisted that John take an extra vacation immediately and promised meanwhile to give him some additional staff to help him.

This case has two lessons: 1. If you feel you're getting out of depth on your job, find out exactly where you stand. Face up to it regardless of the consequences. 2. And if you have a conscientious man like John Jones on your staff, tell him occasionally that you're pleased with his efforts.

You don't have to be a business executive to suffer from excessive tension. I remember a housewife who had always been contented with her home and social life. Now she was "tensed up" all the time and given to unpredictable outbursts of temper. Often she would wander through her house in the middle of the night completely incapable of sleep. A brief discussion revealed that she was worried about the lack of progress of her teenage son, who was more interested in mechanics than in preparing for a law career, as his fond mother wanted. Once she faced up to the fact that both law and industry would be better off if her son headed for mechanical engineering, her symptoms vanished.

Don't Blame the "Rat Race"

Many people who complain of excessive tension brush it off with a reference to the old "rat race"—and obtain a certain perverse pleasure in the illusion that they are working too hard.

I think I can state categorically that few people these days are really working too hard. Rarely do we hear of symptoms that can be traced directly to overwork. Only fifty years ago people worked much longer hours and there were few cases of "tension" and "nerves." Let us recognize that people today spend only 20 per cent of their time at work. The rest of the time—80 per cent—is spent outside the office or shop. More often than not, the causes of excessive tension are to be found in the pattern of life in the nonworking hours.

Sociologists have long been commenting on the problems of leisure time. As a medical man, I can testify that leisure time and "affluence" do produce health problems. Most people are not victims of the rat race. They have created a rat race of their own. They have not learned to deal with their environment.

Because it is easier to ride or drive than walk, most people don't get enough exercise.

Because food and drink are readily available, most people have a weight problem.

Because of built-in entertainment provided by TV, too many people have become passive in their leisure time activities. They do not receive the mental stimulus that active games and lively conversation provide.

Because more and more people travel long distances between home and work, they often neglect their sleep in an effort to spend more time with their families.

In solving the causes of excessive tension, then, it is not enough to examine the job situation. You should examine your whole living pattern to find where you may have strayed.

Establishing Your Tension Threshold

Most people understand their physical limitations. However, many do not seem to realize that the degree of tension one can withstand is highly personal. One person can take a great deal of pressure without an ill effect. The same pressure to another would be incapacitating. If your job or your home environment creates more tension than you can tolerate, don't fight it. Instead, try to change your way of life.

At the same time, you should re-examine your health habits.

In our survey on tension among executives, for instance, this is what we found about the health habits of the 13 per cent who complained of excessive tension.

•When they eat:

they eat breakfast on the fly (under five minutes).

they bolt their lunch (under fifteen minutes).

they hurry through their dinner (under thirty minutes).

and a high percentage are on diets, nursing gastric disorders.

•In their recreation:

few of those complaining of tension get some form of regular exercise.

few have extracurricular interests (church, civic, etc.).

many have no hobby at all.

and one out of five gets no recreation whatsoever.

•For their rest:

many average six or less hours of sleep at night.

few have weekends free for family and self.

and their vacation time is 20 per cent less than the over-all average.

•In their smoking and drinking:

most are heavy cigarette smokers.

most have cocktails for lunch, and many drink more than two.

many have more than two cocktails before dinner.

•In the drugs they take:

most of them use sleep-inducing sedatives.

most of them quiet their nerves with tranquilizers.

If the overly tense person can make a shift in his health habits, this may be all that is needed. If this is not possible, however, then psychiatric help may be indicated.

Conclusions

•We have talked primarily about the persons who already are the victims of excessive stress and tension. These people were not born into the world with these symptoms or, necessarily, with a predisposition to them. Somewhere along the line they acquired habits or failed to face certain situations which brought about these symptoms. If you want to avoid acquiring these symptoms, here are a few guidelines:

•If you have doubts about the ability to do your job well, take steps to find out that you are in the proper line of work, and switch if it seems indicated.

•Face up to the facts of the affluent life and leisure time that most of us now enjoy. Remember that what you do between 9 A.M. and 5 P.M. is not as harmful as what you do between 5 P.M. and 9 A.M.

•Live within your income. Don't worry about "keeping up with the Joneses." This advice may seem out of my field as a physician.

However, we know that conflicts in everyday living build up tension and hence affect your physical well-being.

•If you have trouble getting on with people, socially or on the job, better get some professional help.

•Every desk-bound worker should leave his chair at least once every two hours and walk about the office for a few minutes.

•Chairmen should call for occasional ten-minute intermissions during meetings, breaking up both tension and boredom.

•If you are always tired, you may actually need more physical activity—or you may be bored with what you're doing. Better find out which it is.

•Relaxation in small and large doses is the antidote to excessive tension. This does not mean rest; it means a change of scene, a change of activity.

•The best cure for tension fatigue is exercise, and the best exercise is walking.

•Finally, learn your tension threshold and live within it.

6. That Tired Feeling:
What Can You Do about It?

"Doctor, I'm so tired," is the most common phrase we hear from people day after day. Yet, after we've made a thorough examination, it is rare that we find a physical disorder.

This is not to say that a feeling of constant fatigue is not a danger signal. It is, particularly if it appears suddenly. But I am referring to a kind of chronic, day-in and day-out fatigue, a feeling of tiredness which seems to afflict millions of Americans—and where there is no evidence of disease or of inadequate rest.

I have in mind the person who is tired immediately upon getting out of bed in the morning, the person who attacks his work half-heartedly and then stays in for lunch because "I'm too tired to go out"—the housewife who plans to vacuum the house but doesn't because "I haven't got the strength"—the man who says he has so much to do but maybe he ought to go to bed early to get rested up. There are hundreds of examples of such manifestations of chronic fatigue.

But first let's understand what we mean by fatigue. In its genuine meaning, fatigue is physiological. If we exercise strenuously or work at hard labor, we develop toxic substances in the body. The only antidote is rest for this kind of muscular fatigue.

Illness, such as anemia or thyroid deficiency, can produce fatigue.

But, in the overwhelming number of complaints about fatigue, neither unusual physical exertion nor disease is present. The cause is unknown.

This kind of fatigue is produced in the mind. It is not true fatigue, although to the person it feels like the real article.

There is one basic characteristic of this kind of fatigue. It is boredom.

Boredom: a Plague of the Twentieth Century

This country of ours, the most advanced civilization in history, with the highest standard of living ever known, has produced a generation of bored, apathetic people.

We seek entertainment, yet we find it dull, so that a great performance in the theater is often rewarded by hordes of people rushing out before the curtain falls. We sit in front of TV sets watching a succession of plays, shows, and movies without really noticing what we are seeing. We leaf aimlessly through newspapers and magazines, reading bits and pieces.

When many people say, "I'm tired," they really mean "I'm tired of what I'm doing, I'm tired of my way of life."

We see this attitude in adolescents, who are not fully matured emotionally. I visited friends at their summer place one weekend. Their son, a hulking sixteen-year-old, sat sprawled at the breakfast table. His mother asked him to carry his plate to the kitchen. He moaned piteously and said, "Aw gee, I'm so tired." Five minutes later he was playing football on the beach and continued at high speed hour after hour.

As adults, we laugh at transparency and clearly see that the youth was simply trying to avoid a dull chore and not live up to his family responsibility. It is more difficult for us to realize that many middle-aged persons are guilty of the same ruses and the same immature behavior. And the excuse that is always given is the same: "I'm tired."

A businessman came to me recently with fatigue symptoms. A physical examination revealed that he was in good condition. As we talked over his complaints, he explained that he was "bone weary" from the time he got up in the morning. I learned as we went on that he had built up a successful business, then sold it to a large company at a substantial profit and had a guaranteed income from the company for life as a consultant. He was only forty-five and happily married. I observed that most people would envy him and he blurted out, "They can have it. I'm bored stiff."

I asked him if there was another type of business that interested him. His eyes lit up for the first time and he poured out his ideas for a revolutionary new product. The upshot of it was that he formed a new company, and he called me six months later. "I'm working harder than ever," he said, "and I haven't any idea yet whether this thing will pay off." "It must be very exhausting," I said. "Nonsense," he replied, "I'm never tired anymore." Clearly a new challenge was all this man needed to beat his false fatigue.

An accountant, complaining also of being tired, appeared to me to be a man with no interests outside of his job, which he had long since mastered and it was admittedly routine. When I suggested that he look for outside interests, he was much upset. "I have a great many interests," he said, "more than I can handle. I'm interested in foreign languages, concerts, hi-fi. And I'd like to learn chess if only I had the time." "Tell me," I said, "in the last year have you tried to find time for any of these activities?" Finally he confessed that all he really had done was think about his so-called interests, and maybe he really didn't want to pursue any of them.

This illustrates a point about modern life which we should all understand. Many people with lively imaginations become in-

trigued with the bountiful opportunities for self-improvement—
adult education courses, sports, reading programs, discussion groups.
All of these are made to appear easy to do but upon investigation
require a certain amount of effort. The result is that the person
postpones action but constantly torments himself with guilt feelings
as to the importance of "really getting started."

So don't let yourself be persuaded to undertake hobbies that
you don't genuinely enjoy. If you prefer to walk rather than going
to the golf course, face up to it and relieve your mind. If you
really don't like to take photos, throw away your camera and buy
postcards. You will experience a feeling of relief and your fatigue
may vanish.

Modern Day Hamlets

Every person suffering from boredom fatigue could profit by
rereading *Hamlet,* the classic description of the pitfalls of indecision. Hamlet understood that decisive action was his urgent
need, but he could not bring himself to face the facts. The result was
that he was in a constant mental ferment.

Most bored people do not face the facts about their particular
situations. When brought to the brink of decision, they withdraw
with various excuses such as "There isn't enough time now,"
"Next week will be better," "I'd better rest up and think it
over."

Stretching out a routine job is another way some people avoid
facing the facts. They complain of monotony and blame their jobs
for eating up the time they need to explore more promising fields.
By contrast, I recall reading once about a woman in the French
civil service. She found that she could complete her assigned task
each day in three hours. If she did not turn in her finished work
until the end of the day, she had five hours to herself. Recognizing
this as an opportunity, she proceeded to write a novel, which
launched her on a successful writing career.

How to Clear the Decks for Action

One of my patients told me some years ago how he faced up to his own situation and learned to use action as an antidote for boredom fatigue.

He took the day off, locked himself in his study, and wrote down on paper a list of all the things he had said he would do if there was time. "Do I really want to do this? Am I really interested in this subject?" When the answer was honestly "no," he scratched the item off the list and forgot about it.

He learned many valuable facts about himself. For instance, he had been subscribing to a literary magazine because someone had recommended it. Yet it always went to the bottom of the pile of his business magazines, which he usually read thoroughly. So he faced the fact that he really enjoyed business subjects and that literary subjects were not his cup of tea. He cancelled the subscription. He learned that he had been avoiding playing golf at his new club, and that the real reason was that golf made him irritable and that he hated the long trip out of the city. So he resigned and joined a city club where he could play squash and swim.

Having faced up to the facts about himself, he felt renewed and no longer suffered from fatigue.

A Nation of Worriers

A recent survey by public opinion analyst Louis Harris revealed that a high proportion of Americans are much concerned about personal failings such as eating too much, being out of shape physically, not reading enough, wasting too much time. In fact, he says, worries about such personal failings beset some of the population almost all of the time.

Most significant, I thought, was his observation that the principal worriers are college-educated, upper income professionals and executives, while the people who worry least are farmers. Farmers, of course, are physically active, and they experience genuine, not imaginary, fatigue at the end of each day. The professional and executive groups live principally in their minds; they can't keep up with all that they want to do, and, as our own experience confirms, they are not physically active enough.

The "Tireless" Person

Let's reverse the coin for a moment. Instead of dwelling on the tired person let's look at those people we all know who seem to be "tireless." I think, for example, of a onetime neighbor of mine, a woman with six children, who was always seeking new things to do "to fill the time." One obvious characteristic was that she was always on the move, always interested and challenged by whatever she was doing, in other words, the opposite of bored.

And I think of an executive I saw regularly over the years. He would seem to have his hands full because he ran one of the largest companies in the country. Yet he always appeared to have enough time to play squash each day and to collect books, in which field he was a recognized expert. He never complained about being tired or worried. The answer, he told me, was organizing his time, picking hobbies he enjoyed. For example, he accepted the chairmanship of the community fund drive. But, instead of making it an extra duty, and hence being so overloaded that he wouldn't do a good job for either the fund or his company, he arranged for his executive vice-president to assume some of his duties during the fund drive. "After all," he said, "there are only the same number of hours each day. It is impossible, if those hours are already committed, to get additional hours. Further, I'll retire someday and I'd like my replacement to start getting some direct experience."

The point is that these "tireless" types concentrate hard on whatever they are doing—plan their time—and hence have no vacant periods in which they churn about trying to decide what to do next. Maybe these people were born with a little more energy than the rest of us, but I doubt it. They're simply better managers of their time and they don't suffer from the Hamlet complex.

Some Steps to Overcome Fatigue

We've stated the problem. Now, what can you do if you are a victim of chronic fatigue? Here are some steps that may help:

1. Have a complete physical examination. The odds are heavily in your favor that there will be no physical disorder present. Probably, at the most, 5 per cent examined for this complaint will require physical treatment. But you should have the examination to reassure yourself and to understand your condition.

2. Examine your daily routine. List your activities on paper, exactly how you spend your time. Then, on a separate sheet, write down the things you say you want to do but never get around to. Ask yourself, do you really want to do these things? If "deep in your heart" you know you have no real interest in learning French or taking guitar lessons, forget it. You'll find a burden lifted almost immediately.

On the other hand, if your problem is that you can't find anything that really interests you, start to ask yourself why not. Perhaps, you'll find, you'd like to take up a hobby, like photography, but you hesitate because you don't know the techniques and you think you are "too old." Just remember, you're never too old until you're dead. Now I wouldn't recommend that a forty-year-old man suddenly take up football, but there are plenty of sports and other activities where there's always time to get started. A friend of mine is devoted to horseback riding, yet, as I learned recently, he'd never been on a horse until his fiftieth birthday. He'll never win any competitions, but he enjoys his daily canter and it gives zest to his life.

3. Zest! That's a key word in overcoming that tired feeling. People who are not tired are enthusiastic and optimistic, the contrary of the always fatigued person. Once I mentioned this to a patient, however, and he rebuked me. "How can I feel enthusiastic when the world is in such a terrible situation, our crime rate is rising, people are living in misery in our slums, our hospitals are inadequately staffed?" My reply was another question. "Isn't there something you could do about it?" We talked further and we located a hospital nearby that badly needed a volunteer to run an entertainment program. My friend took over the post on a trial basis. Now, five years later, he pours his energies—with enthusiasm—into this new-found interest, an interest he had all along but he didn't know how to get started.

4. Avoid loneliness. Many chronic-fatigued persons live too much with themselves.

5. Plan your days so that you have pleasant events to look forward to. If you're in a routine job, have your evening planned in advance. Anticipation is one of the pleasures of life.

6. Avoid the fallacy of excessive rest. Bored, always tired people often go to bed earlier than they need in order to, as they say, "rest up." If there is no physical disorder, then extra rest will do nothing to eliminate the feeling of fatigue. It will still be there in the morning.

7. Take an interest in other people. If you are always tired, it helps to talk over your situation with someone else. Your doctor would like to hear your story, but he's too busy with truly sick patients. Your minister, who is there to counsel you, is also overworked these days. So the easiest solution is simply to talk to a friend. You might start by asking him if he's always tired. Regardless of which way he answers, you'll begin to forget yourself—and that's the first step to recovery.

In looking back, I realize that I'm talking about living habits and not medicine. The reason is that we're discussing health, and the maintenance of health is a job for you, and not your doctor. In fact, the great proportion of complaints brought to the medical profession are not physical in origin, and there's no treatment available.

Conclusions

*Chronic fatigue—"that tired feeling"—is an increasingly common complaint.

*Extra rest will not cure it.

*Drugs and pills and energy medicine and vitamins will not improve the condition.

*The root of chronic fatigue is boredom, a product of our affluent society, where the material goods are easy to come by. Or, in case of the underprivileged, where there is a complete lack of hope for the future. Either way, it produces apathetic people.

*The chances are remote that constant fatigue is physical in origin. But, to make sure, have a thorough physical examination. Because if your fatigue appears suddenly, it could be a danger signal.

*If your doctor pronounces you physically fit, then examine your daily living routine. Make sure that you have things to do that interest you, and interest yourself in the people around you. Be enthusiastic. Avoid adding more to your schedule than you can actually handle.

*Step up your physical activity. Increased leisure time is a hazard unless we get sufficient exercise. The sedentary routine of modern work requires that we ourselves seek the physical activity our bodies require. We can no longer get sufficient exercise from our jobs.

*If you have more things you think you'd like to do but never even start to do, dismiss them from your mind. Or, if you can't think of anything you'd like to do, force yourself to learn a new skill and shortly you will find that you enjoy it.

•You are never too old to learn a new game or sport or hobby.

•Try to be decisive. Life is full of choices that must be faced daily. Reread *Hamlet* to understand the tragedy that indecision can bring.

•And, if you feel yourself overwhelmed and concerned about the miseries of today's world, try to do something in your own way about the situation. Remember what Emerson said: "This is the best of all possible times to be alive if we but knew it."

7. Who Needs Sleep?
What You Should Know
about Sleep and Rest

If someone offered you a formula for longer life, general well-being, energy, and instant relief from fatigue and tension, how much would it be worth to you? If I could put the formula in a bottle, doubtless millions of people would buy it.

But the formula I have in mind is free to all. It is sleep—and in our hectic modern age it is often neglected or misunderstood. In fact, it sometimes seems to me that the more knowledge we acquire the more we forget about the simple fundamentals. Sleep is one of those fundamentals of good health where many of us need a "refresher" course.

Life begins with sleep. Insomnia in an infant is unheard of. The baby, the child, the adolescent need a great deal of sleep. And if the habits of sleep in the growing-up years are allowed to develop naturally, the adult will not be troubled with difficulty in sleeping.

It is in the tacit recognition of the unusual requirements for sleep in the young that we sometimes get off base. Youngsters equate staying up late with maturity. They falsely reason that the less sleep they have the more they are getting a head start on becoming an adult. Actually, they are setting a pattern which will handicap them the rest of their lives. They will develop into the kind of person who brags about how little sleep he gets, then begins to fret about his inability to sleep, and another insomniac has been created.

Man's inquiring and restless nature leads him persistently to try to beat the game. The warlike Aztecs, in the bloodiest of battles, never thought of fighting at night, and neither did their opponents. Night was for sleeping. The ambitious Cortez "broke the rules" through his night attacks, and in modern warfare long periods without sleep are accepted as part of the routine. The excitement of present day business and politics also produces a climate where attempts are made to beat the game. But we are still limited by a twenty-four-hour day where the rules of the "health game" have not changed—and are not likely to change—despite such marvels as the conquest of outer space, computers, and automation.

Since you're not going to get out of the world alive, you might as well learn how to live in it. And sleep has a definite function in both how you feel from day to day and how you live out your full years.

The Nature of Sleep

The exact mechanism by which the body produces sleep is not yet known, despite numerous research studies. However, the important consideration here is understanding the effects of sleep on the body and on the brain.

The body needs to be completely idle for a sufficient length of time to permit the elimination of waste products. When we are active during the day, the constant contractions of our muscles produce certain chemicals that normally are disposed of as waste. But, while we are active, the rate of disposal is not sufficient to prevent fatigue. It is thought, therefore, that, as this fatigue builds up, sleep results.

Regardless, we know that after adequate sleep the body is as good as new. And conversely, without enough sleep, there is still the feeling of fatigue because not all of the waste has been eliminated.

The day's activities also produce an incredible number of sensations on the brain. If we had no relief from this barrage, some authorities believe that we would all become psychotic. The safeguard of sanity and the relief from the stress of millions of sensory impulses come from sleep.

However, there is no such thing as completely "sound" sleep in which we are totally detached from our senses. The first stage of sleep comes within the first hour or so after we go to bed. Gradually we lose our flow of thoughts and become detached from the world about us. A sound or flash of light will awaken us.

The next phase carries us into deeper sleep, much of it dreamless. Even so, a shaking hand on the shoulder, a light in the eyes, an alarm clock can awaken us.

The final phase of sleep comes early in the morning when sleep tends to lighten. There are no sharply defined lines between the various stages of sleep. Some persons take longer than others to move from stage to stage. However, we should understand something about the basic mechanism in order to understand how to overcome difficulties in sleeping.

Why Sleep Is Important

We have seen that there are two kinds of fatigue, body fatigue and brain fatigue. Whatever your activity, therefore, you experience fatigue, and if deprived of sleep you are robbed of a sense of well-being. Think back to the last restless night you had. How did you feel the next day? Could you think as well, could you follow conversations, did you do as much work, did you feel life was a joy or a bore? The chances are that you were overly fatigued and this came about because of lack of sleep.

Should you still doubt the effects of inadequate sleep, consider some experiments that have been made. Studies at the Walter Reed Army Institute of Research, in Washington, have shown that the longest a person can go without sleep is 240 hours. And the volunteers who went through these routines found the experience akin to torture. Measurements of the physiological results revealed numerous harmful effects. Most significant was the damage to the brain. After some sixty-five hours of sleeplessness, one human guinea pig was found in a washroom. He was frantically trying to wash away the cobwebs which he said covered his face. The results of these experiments tend to demonstrate strongly that sleep is essential for the maintenance of emotional stability, if not complete sanity.

Myths about Sleep

For something that is so natural and built-in as sleep, there are an amazing number of myths and misconceptions still prevalent. Here are a few of them:

Myth: An hour of sleep before midnight is worth two hours after midnight.

Fact: This myth overlooks the two basic kinds of sleeping habits, which Sir William Osler once labeled as "owls" and "larks." Some people, like owls, prefer to work late and get up late; we often refer to this type as a "night person." Others, the larks, get up early in the morning and retire early. Whichever you are, it makes no difference, provided that you get the right amounts of sleep. And this is the same whether you are an owl or a lark.

Myth: Four or five hours of sound sleep are worth more than eight or ten hours of restless slumber.

Fact: There is no substitute for the total number of hours of sleep required. While it is best to sleep soundly, the important point is to sleep the minimum number of hours, seven or eight.

Myth: Your eight hours of sleep each day should be consecutive, not broken up.

Fact: It is perfectly satisfactory to break up your periods of sleep. Many people, Edison being the most famous, sleep a few hours at night and take frequent naps during the day. This is particularly true in the entertainment world. Yet for those with this practice, most suffer no ill effects.

Myth: You can get your sleep just as well by cat-napping in a chair as by lying in bed.

Fact: Resting in bed is much more satisfactory than sleeping in a chair. Horizontal sleep is of a better quality, as I think anyone who ever tried to sleep overnight in an airplane will testify.

What Happens if You Don't Sleep Enough?

Many talented, ambitious people seek ways to cut down on their sleep because they are anxious to gain extra hours for their particular interests. I recall a young businessman who used to ask me for research studies about sleep. I soon learned that he was trying to find out if science had any suggestions for getting as much sleep out of four hours as out of eight hours. I assured him that this was unlikely and that he ought to realize that he was just the same as the rest of us in his need for regular rest. He persisted, however, and kept cutting back his sleep in his desire to have more waking moments. One day he came down with tuberculosis. His resistance was so low that he needed to take off six months from his job for complete rest. All the time that he thought he had gained was immediately wiped out, and he was fortunate that he made a full recovery.

Short-changing yourself on sleep may not catch up with you for many years. But it will catch up. One inevitable day you will "suddenly" lose your energy, become prone to various ailments, and find your general health rapidly deteriorating.

Sleep and Longevity

On the basis of our Life Extension examinations over the years and other studies I have seen, I am completely convinced that sleep and longevity are directly related. I believe that the effects of sleeplessness are cumulative and that the damage to your health is permanent and irreversible. It is perhaps no accident that many family doctors do not live out their normal life spans, for so many of them go week after week on far less sleep than people in other walks of life.

If sleep has rejuvenating powers, it should be clear that the lack of sleep will make our bodies more vulnerable to disease. As Dr. Edmund Jacobson, director of the Chicago Laboratory for Clinical Psychology, has said: "The effects of inadequate sleep are hard to measure: a little less zeal and ambition, an extra cold, or perhaps a more serious disease which might have passed you by . . ." And Dr. E. Cuyler Hammond has made studies which show that those who average seven to eight hours of sleep have the best life expectancy.

Can You "Make Up" Sleep?

Suppose you get home late from the theater and, instead of your regular eight hours of sleep, you only get five hours. Chances are that you will feel the effects all the next day. But will you need to sleep eleven hours the next night to make up for the three you lost the night before?

Normally not. Usually if you get back on your schedule and have your regular eight hours, you will feel just as good as usual the following day. Just the same, the loss of that sleep can have a cumulative effect. If week after week, month after month, you have frequent periods of this practice, you will get yourself hopelessly in debt, and no amount of "making up" will be possible. The damage will have been done.

Yet one of the remarkable things about the human organism is that it is never too late to change your schedule. If you get back on an eight-hour sleep basis regularly, your health and well-being will improve.

Sleep and Your Emotional Health

Some people who are consistently short on sleep by an hour or so each day develop emotional disorders. I remember an executive who kept complaining about his feelings of constant anxiety. When he came to tell me about it, he asked whether he should go to a psychiatrist. I queried him about his sleep patterns. He told me, "I get maybe five or six hours a night, sometimes less. But I really don't need any more." When I advised him to get more sleep, he balked, saying that he couldn't sleep more if he wanted to. A hacking cough made his sleep fitful. His cough was obviously due to cigarette smoking, three packs a day. He agreed to stop his smoking and try to get more sleep.

He tells me that his cough has gone, he sleeps his full eight hours, gets more work done, and is amazed to think he had ever thought of going to a psychiatrist.

Dr. Henry O. Laughlin, a professor of psychiatric medicine, has studied "The Role of Sleep in Emotional Health." According to Dr. Laughlin, "Were it not for the benefit of sleep, the cumulative effects of even the usual stresses and strains of our daily life could be overwhelming."

For those who have learned to use the power of sleep, it can be amazingly effective in moments of emotional crisis.

I was away on a trip when a friend of mine, an elderly gentleman, went through the grueling experience of the funeral of his wife of fifty-five years. When I returned I spoke to his daughter and expressed my regret that I had not been on hand to perhaps give him a sedative to see him through the ordeal. She said, "He's done better than any of us. He went to bed right after dinner, slept through the night, and is in top flight shape."

Your own bed can keep you off the psychiatrist's couch.

Can You Sleep Too Much?

Normally our concern is with people who don't sleep enough. However, there are some people who sleep regularly much more than the norm—ten to twelve hours. Sometimes these are people suffering from some organic disorder. More often than not, however, such people are simply bored and in their waking hours have less vigor and take less interest in life than the rest of us.

The real test for the correct amount of sleep, however, is how well you feel each day, how well you do your work, your general sense of well-being and fitness. Many people who go through life without enough sleep have forgotten how it feels to have a normal sense of well-being. They sometimes have to go through a long illness where they are forced to stay in bed and learn how to sleep before they regain the sleep habit.

Insomnia: No One Ever Died of It, but . . .

There is no such person as a true "insomniac." As we have seen in reviewing the mechanisms of sleep, it is impossible to stay awake indefinitely without falling asleep. There is no question however, that far too many people these days have difficulty in getting to sleep, or in remaining asleep during the night.

The causes are seldom organic. Rather the enemies of sleep are excessive fatigue, worry, tension, and false personal attitudes toward sleep.

"Sleep is a waste of time. I have so much to do," one of my patients once said, adding, "After all, I'll be dead a long time."

"Wrong," I replied. "You'll be dead a lot longer."

If you have lost the built-in sleep habit you inherited when you entered the world, you must take a "refresher course" in learning to sleep. Here are a few suggestions to follow:

1. Try to keep your hours of sleep as regular as possible. Find out which hours are best for you. Try various schedules until you get the right one. As soon as you start getting up each morning feeling refreshed, you'll know that you have the right pattern.

2. Sleep in a dark and quiet room.

3. Make every effort to relax your body physically. A brief walk or some other moderate exercise may do the trick. Sometimes a warm bath is helpful. The whole idea is to make your going-to-bed time a fixed but relaxed routine. Don't try to force yourself to sleep. This is going to have the opposite effect.

4. Make sure you have a comfortable bed and mattress. For some curious reason the American double bed is actually smaller than two single beds put together. If you are a large person and prefer a double bed, perhaps one of the new king-sized beds is for you.

5. Keep the room cool but not necessarily cold. Don't worry about whether you have several windows wide open. The important thing is that the temperature is right for you.

6. Avoid excessive stimulation late in the day. Stay away from competitive sports, avoid nighttime arguments. Reading is usually better than TV just before retirement because it is less stimulating.

7. If you must have a drink before bed, stick to warm milk. Tea and coffee contain caffeine, which tends to stimulate.

8. Try to prepare for sleep by slowing down at least an hour before getting into bed. Dr. Dean Foster, consultant to the Sleep Research Foundation, once wrote, "Going to sleep is like stopping a car at an intersection. A driver who sees a traffic light change a block away is better off slowing down gradually and coasting to a stop, rather than coming to a sudden brake-slamming halt."

9. Don't count sheep. Like muscular effort, mental activity while lying in bed can interfere with sleep.

10. Remember that lying quietly in bed for several hours, even though sleep does not come, is better than getting up and fussing around the house.

Should You Use Sleeping Pills?

Normally one doesn't need sleeping pills, but, if used, they should be under the direction of your physician. Sleeping pills are simply a crutch. If employed too regularly, you will develop a tolerance for them, and then they lose their effectiveness.

However, sedatives can be used if you are trying to regain your normal habits of sleep. Here is such a routine, which I recommend:

1. Take the pill three nights in succession.

2. On the fourth night, put the pill on a nearby table and try to forget it's there. If sleep does not come after a reasonable time, then take the pill.

3. Repeat Step Two every night until you find that you have fallen asleep without the pill. If meantime you have been following the other suggestions for sleep which I mentioned earlier, a new habit will take over, and sleep will become easier.

Conclusions

• Despite the space age and the marvelous achievements of science, we have the same physical limitations of our ancestors. This means, for most people, about eight hours of sleep each day.

• Sleep not only restores our physical energy, it preserves our sanity and emotional health.

• The sleep habit is built into us as infants. No infant ever has insomnia. It is never too late to regain the sleep habit.

• If you prefer a poetic approach to sleep. I recommend that you keep in your bedroom the following quotation from Cervantes' *Don Quixote:*

"Now blessings light on him that first invented this same sleep! It covers a man all over, thoughts and all, like a cloak; 'tis meat for the hungry, drink for the thirsty, heat for the cold, and cold for the hot. 'Tis the current coin that purchases all the pleasures of the world cheap; and the balance that sets the king and the shepherd, the fool and the wise man even."

It is still true today.

8. The Use of Leisure Time: a Health Opportunity

The tremendous increase in leisure time—and the promise of more to come—should make us the healthiest people in history. Yet this is not so. In fact, there is ample evidence that leisure time and affluence may in large measure be responsible for the upsurge in degenerative diseases such as coronary heart disease.

Leisure time, the shorter work week, and automation are often discussed from the points of view of business, labor, the economy, and our social structure. It is time that we examined the health consequences as well.

Science and technology have placed us on the verge of a revolutionary way of life in which machines and computers will take over much of the world's work. Getting rid of the drudgery and making one's living with less and less physical effort are an appealing prospect. But unless we adopt an equally revolutionary approach to our use of this new leisure time, we may wipe out the gains that medicine has won for us over the past century.

Leisure time, wisely used, can be beneficial to the health. It is not a one-way street, however. Drastic changes in our pattern of living may be called for.

In order to point out the opportunities of lesiure time for those who want a longer and happier life, let us trace briefly the rise of leisure time over the past fifty years or so.

Not so long ago the twelve-hour workday was commonplace. And even with the eight-hour day, half days of work on Saturday were standard until a decade or so ago. Nowadays, the schedule has shifted so that we spend only 20 per cent of our time on the job.

Just the same, for most working people excessive leisure time is more an illusion than a reality. But already most of us are leisure-oriented and more of our time and thinking go into our personal activities. More and more we worry and plan how to make the most of our own time.

A Typical Schedule

Let's look at the hours involved in a typical schedule to see what's happening.

If you work eight hours (including lunch) and sleep eight hours, you have eight hours daily of so-called leisure time. And you have sixteen additional hours on Saturday and Sunday.

What has to come out of your own time?

_____Eating

_____Personal Hygiene

_____Going to and from work

_____Shopping

_____Civic and organizational meetings

_____Recreation, such as sports, theater, concerts, reading, cards, TV, radio, hobbies, your family

The proportion of time you spend on each and the way you handle these activities can have a profound effect on your health.

It is in the so-called recreation area where the temptations are the greatest. The opportunities for recreation are so easy, so varied, so appealing that some people find that they can't be contained in even eight hours of free time.

It is not, for most employed people, a problem to do something; it is what to do out of many choices. And some people become like the child who won't leave his toys to come to dinner.

So it is not leisure time that affects us; it is the nature of the leisure time activities.

In many cases eight hours is not enough, and infringements are made on the rest of the time.

Sleep is one. By no means all of the people watching the *Late Late Show* are unemployed or retired. They are people who have to be on the job at eight-thirty or nine. And when they come dragging in, eating a Danish at the desk, they are now beginning to cut into the work time as well.

Perhaps the greatest block of time available—unprecedented in history—is the modern weekend. From 5 P.M. Friday to 9 A.M. Monday is sixty-four hours—sixty-four hours of freedom from the job. And most people crowd everything they can into those sixty-four hours. Trips are a great favorite and many people travel hundreds of miles and stay up later than usual, thus making blue Monday a national institution.

How Leisure Time Affects Health

So it is what is being done in leisure time, and what is being borrowed in addition from the sleep and work segments of the day, that has such a bearing on the health.

If you will jot down the amount of time you spend on recreational eating, recreational drinking, recreational smoking, and other passive activities—as well as how much you short yourself on sleep— you will begin to understand the problem. Leisure time is healthful. What takes place in your leisure time is not necessarily so.

The main factor, regardless of what you do, is whether it is active or passive, physical or not physical.

To understand what has happened, and why we are concerned about it from a health point of view, let us take a long look backward. At the beginning of this nation we were largely a rural people. A man lived by physical effort. Later, as we industrialized, a man still had a good deal of physical activity at his job. Our ancestors, in their brief leisure time, were completely entitled to flop down by the fire and do nothing. They kept in physical trim through the rigors of their occupations.

But today—and it will be more so in the coming computer age— fewer and fewer people derive any physical activity from their jobs. And if the body does not have enough exercise, it will deteriorate.

Our work routines are largely sedentary. We ride from door to door if we possibly can. We sit at desks and machines. We patronize the nearest restaurant. And, having barely moved our bodies for eight to ten hours, we go home to sit in front of our TV sets. After five days of sitting we feel so exhausted that we spend the weekend resting!

In our periodic health examinations we find far too many sad examples of this kind of passive living. And, in simple terms, this may be one reason why we are finding that degenerative diseases, such as heart disease, are taking such a heavy toll.

The issue is, then, can we learn to switch our periods of physical activity from our work time to our leisure time? For if we do not, the health problems will become formidable indeed.

Needed: "Active" Leisure Time Activities

Out of your leisure time must come a program of regular physical activity. Of course you should enjoy the abundance of pleasures our civilization offers: radio, TV, stamp collecting, cards, photography, reading, concerts, the theater. But if your bent is toward these passive types of activity, you must then build into your leisure time a suitable proportion of pastimes that are physically active in nature.

This bring us to sports, the kind that lend themselves to lifetime and regular use. Highly competitive, strenuous sports are fine for young people, but we are thinking now primarily of the great middle-aged group, where the health problems are also greatest.

Suitable sports of this group are bicycling, swimming, bowling, fencing, horseback riding, table tennis, golf. It is important, then, that you see that your children learn one or more of these lifetime sports so that they become proficient enough to want to continue them in their adult lives.

There are other recreational activities such as roller skating, ice skating, and dancing which also provide good exercise. I include in dancing, incidentally, folk dances and square dances, which I believe should be encouraged. Ironically, these dances originated with rural people who got plenty of exercise through a long day's hard work, yet who still sought this strenuous type of relaxation. This simply proves that the more the body is exercised the more exercise is enjoyed. But the out-of-condition person finds it painful to walk to the corner drugstore to buy aspirin.

Social critics have long deplored our tendency toward spectator sports in this country. From a health point of view, I also deplore the tendency. At the least, try to get out to the ball park rather than doing all your observing on TV.

A by-product of active use of leisure time is that you can work off frustrations and tensions that develop in sedentary types of work. Any exercise that provides brisk movement, gets the circulation going, has a refreshing effect, rather than being tiring.

Relieving Tension and Fatigue

Recently I read some tips on making speeches by a business executive recognized for his proficiency. He pointed out that, if you work hard at delivering a speech, you will have built up an emotional charge. This, plus the strain of facing a strange audience, may leave you weak-kneed and with a slight headache once the speech is over. And then he proceeded to tell, out of his own experience, the formula for getting rid of the symptoms. "Do not," he said, "take a taxi to the station or your hotel or back to the office. Simply get outside and walk vigorously for half an hour."

I wish more people realized that the way to relieve a feeling of mental fatigue is not to sit, but to get some physical exercise.

The Importance of Walking

By this time you should know that I am prejudiced in favor of walking, and that I stress it as the single most important exercise available. The point about walking is that it can be fitted into any kind of routine, no special equipment is necessary, you can set your own pace, you don't need teammates, and you can practice it daily. So put walking at the top of your list of regular leisure time activities.

Some people object to walking because they say it's dull. This is not so if you use your eyes. If you look at the amazing assortment of people you encounter—the shopwindows, the houses, the trees and shrubbery—you will quickly "forget" you're walking, and you'll be mentally refreshed.

A young real estate agent told me recently how he uses leisure time walking to increase his knowledge of buildings in the city. When the streets are not crowded, he wanders through the business area, looking up toward the tops of the buildings. In so doing, he finds, the buildings no longer look alike. They assume personalities and characteristics of their own. And he has learned that the buildings have architectural features and decorations that he had never noticed before—in fact, that most people never see because they walk with their heads down. So walking for him has now become the pursuit of a hobby—architectural design—and this is the way it should be. Every leisure time activity should have an element of adventure or fun.

What about Vacations and Long Weekends?

Vacations are essential and more people than ever before have them. Long weekends, combined with holidays, are more prevalent. Admittedly, getting away from home is certainly good for anyone. But if your vacations are simply longer periods of more food, more drinking, more sitting, this is self-defeating. And if your daily routine does not provide regular exercise, you won't be in condition to do the walking that one must encounter in any kind of travel.

Once again, then, we stress establishing a daily pattern of good use of leisure time, and not just vacations and weekends.

A Positive Approach to Leisure Time

How can you set up the kind of routine I have been discussing? How can you fit in enough regular activity into your daily life?

First, go back over your schedule once more and learn how much time you have away from the job. Figure out how much time you need for traveling back and forth to work, how much for meals, and be sure not to touch your eight hours for sleep.

Somewhere in this you can certainly fit in an hour for walking. It doesn't have to be at one single period. Perhaps you can arrange to walk twenty minutes in the morning and twenty minutes at night as you go to and from work. And you certainly can pick a restaurant ten minutes away, which will give you twenty minutes of walking at noon. When the weather is good, a walk after dinner or just before bedtime is possible for most people.

This would give you the minimum you need. But there are other possibilities. Select a sport that you can participate in not only on weekends, but during the week. More and more swimming pools are becoming available. A swim at the end of the day is wonderfully refreshing. By cutting down on your cocktail period, you can find the time for this. And we have mentioned other active recreations, such as dancing, or table tennis, which most people find enjoyable.

There are still other possibilities. Try a few setting-up exercises each morning, not strenuous calisthenics, but things you can do as you are getting dressed. Again, many people find that even ten minutes of calisthenics are boring. But if you take a shower, you can do a few exercises at the same time. As you are washing your face, you can do a few knee bends. And as you walk around your bedroom, you can stretch and bend. These routines will not take extra time, but they will be richly rewarding in health dividends.

Even though your job may be confining, you can doubtless find ways to take an occasional exercise break, again just doing simple, nonstrenuous exercises. I have long advocated that business firms install a small recreation room on the executive floor where a man can drive a golf ball or ride a bicycle for a few minutes several times a day.

Industry wisely recognizes that its most valuable asset is its employees. It provides more and more benefits, including so-called health insurance, which is really accident and sickness insurance. Industry could do itself and its employees a service by providing athletic clubs and perhaps a swimming pool, just as many provide a company cafeteria. We should encourage exercise breaks as well.

We need new types of games that induce action. A well-deserved fortune awaits the person who invents an appealing game that can be played on a space the size of a bridge table, and that requires physical effort to play it.

On weekends, continue your quest for active recreation. Don't loaf around all day in a bathrobe. Get dressed and get out on both Saturday and Sunday. To succeed at this, you will have to plan projects that will force you to be active. When did you last visit your local museum? It's full of fascinating displays, and it makes for good walking. Imagine yourself in a foreign city on a weekend. Would you stay in your hotel room? Of course not, you'd go out to see the sights. Have you seen all the sights yet in your city? I doubt it.

An Amazing Coincidence

Two men who died a while ago on the same day epitomized in the extreme the best and the worst in health habits. One man was Farouk, former King of Egypt, the other Amos Alonzo Stagg, the football coach (and active in Life Extension Institute in its initial year, 1914). Stagg didn't drink or smoke. He coached football until he was in his nineties, operated a hand lawn mower until he was ninety-eight, and lived to be 102. Farouk indulged in every known excess, never worked, weighed three hundred pounds, and died at forty-five.

Perhaps few of us can practice our health habits as rigorously as did Stagg, and some may say that if they followed his regimen there would be no fun in living to be 102. But how can one say that a three-hundred-pound man with multiple ailments in his best years had fun? Seldom have we seen such dramatic evidence of the fact that good health lies in moderation.

Conclusions

•To take full advantage of your leisure time, you need to know how you are now spending your days.
•When you have added up the time on your job, traveling back and forth to work, your meals, and eight hours of sleep, the balance is what you have for your own use.
•There are more and more tempting ways to spend your time, and you have freedom of choice. My advice is, however, that you seek out active recreations, rather than passive ones.
•Old-fashioned thinking? Well, the human body is an old-fashioned machine, too. Until we get a new model, we'll have to use the same rules regardless of how much or how little leisure time we have.

9. A Word about Pill Taking— a National Pastime

In the many ways in which our country leads the world, pill taking is surely near the top. And vitamins, pep pills, and tranquilizers are high on the list of items consumed.

In the case of vitamins, no damage is done except to the pocketbook. As to pep pills and tranquilizers, their unauthorized use can be dangerous. Frequently we read in the papers about a new tranquilizer being withdrawn from the market because of harmful side effects. Mind you, the drug manufacturer had carefully tested the product for perhaps years, yet there were still unknown patterns that no one suspected. Small wonder that doctors are cautious in prescribing tranquilizers. Yet many laymen dose themselves frequently with no thought of the consequences.

The average person has no need for all of this pill swallowing. If you eat normally, you need no supplements. You get your vitamins from your food. If you get enough rest and exercise, you need nothing to "pep you up." And if you are reasonably happy at home and office, there is no need to suppress your emotions through tranquilizers.

Aren't there any times when the use of these pills is justified?

Of course, but under very special circumstances which we shall describe and only upon a physician's advice. Self-medication for real or fancied ills is a dubious practice at best. It can be a lethal pastime when the taker indiscriminately swallows excessive quantities of drugs.

The Perils of Pep Pills

Pep pills are far from harmless—in fact, they're becoming a major menace. Known also as "goof balls," they have been responsible for crimes, accidents, and tragic deaths, particularly among many teenagers. The police are constantly uncovering illegal supplies and confiscating them because of these effects. But because they appeal to man's burning desire to acquire unlimited strength and energy (or at least the illusion) pep pills are consumed in sensational amounts. Despite the fact that most states forbid their sales except when prescribed, enough pills are produced annually to supply every person in the country with more than twenty each!

There are, naturally, certain beneficial uses of pep pills in the treatment of disease. People suffering from emotional depressions or incurable illnesses are helped immensely by the "lift" which the pep pill can give. Elderly people, too, often find life more enjoyable if they can augment their fading energy. Any possible harmful effects are outbalanced by a richer life for such persons in the twilight years. But even in these cases, they should be prescribed only under a doctor's direction.

There have been times also when I have prescribed these pills for a busy executive who is working overtime to get out an important report or who has a temporary need to be unusually alert. But these are rare occasions. The continued use of such an internal crutch will not improve performance, increase strength, or add to your normal supply of energy.

Pep pills produce delusions. Upon taking one a person feels stimulated and invigorated. Actually, the pill covers up natural physiological tiredness. As one goes on, there develops a feeling of restlessness and tenseness, even sleeplessness. But the dangerous effect is the letdown that most people experience when the drug wears off. If the drug is used to prevent sleep while driving, the letdown comes without warning. Overpowering fatigue follows and a far greater hazard is involved. Another hazard in taking any drug that terminates in depression is the ease with which it leads to the twin evils of habituation and overdosage. When the effect wears off, the temptation is great to repeat the dose and frequently larger doses are needed.

Pep pills cannot prevent fatigue; they merely obscure its recognition. Such a process may lead to immoderation and place a heavy strain on the heart and circulatory system. One wants to "keep going," not go to sleep. Thus fatigue, the best warning signal we have to stop, rest, and rebuild, is suppressed. This should not be allowed to happen. A feeling of premature fatigue tells us that something is wrong. If the day's work becomes increasingly harder to finish and the balance is not restored by sleep, a thorough physical checkup is needed—not pills.

The only long-term solution to unnatural fatigue is improving the physical equipment. Revalue your activities. Drop unnecessary business entertainment. Precondition yourself for extra efforts by walking more, sleeping more, eating sensibly, cutting down on alcohol and smoking. If you will build up your natural reserve of energy, it will see you through emergencies that no pill can handle.

One other aspect of pep pills should be mentioned. When they were first introduced, it was noted that they curtailed the appetite. Some doctors experimented with them in treating patients for overweight. The difficulty was that the additional effect of overstimulation affected the sleep patterns of these patients. So in weight control, too, pep pills are not effective. Because like all appetite depressants, when they are stopped, the appetite returns and the weight goes back up.

In short, the great majority of normal healthy people can go a lifetime without ever needing a single pep pill.

Tranquilizers: Taming the Tiger in You

Where pep pills give you the illusion of unleashing the "tiger in the tank," tranquilizers put the lid on. And some people do it just that way. Having built up so much tension from pep pills that they can't sleep, they then resort to tranquilizers. The result is often a swing too far in the other direction, giving the person a feeling of living on a roller coaster.

Tranquilizers, too, have a recognized position in medicine, but they are definitely not for self-prescription. Tranquilizers are simply a newer form of sedative, replacing in some cases the older barbiturates. Their primary purpose is in the treatment of emotionally disturbed psychiatric patients. Tranquilizers can calm exaggerated reactions so that the need for institutional care is minimized, often eliminated. Their use for normal persons is extremely limited. When a person is awaiting surgery or under some short-term emotional stress, the doctor may well prescribe a tranquilizer. But to use them to relieve everyday stress and strain and conflict is to use a sledge hammer on a thumbtack.

Tranquilizers are not new discoveries. Only the name is new and its selection was a ten strike as a sales promotion device. The very name lulls people into feeling that these pills can only be good for you. Yet these are potent drugs and far from harmless. They have gotten into the folklore of Madison Avenue along with the ulcer as a typical habit of the hard-driving, stress-ridden advertising executive. Actually, a creative person in particular should avoid curbing his emotions through a drug. Without a certain amount of pressure and obstacles talented people cannot rise to the heights. It is facing up to challenge that produces great accomplishments.

Emotional stamina is present in each of us, and at intervals it will be tested. The emotionally mature person will seldom need a tranquilizer to meet such tests. And most certainly the competitive executive should not require medication to cushion his ordinary business responsibilities. If he does, it is an admission that he is unable to cope.

Tranquilizers when used by normal people provide a release from reality. In that sense, alcohol is still the Number One tranquilizer—its use as old as man. Yet no one has ever seriously recommended alcohol as a psychotherapeutic agent to be used every time the going becomes a little rough.

Sedatives, such as tranquilizers and alcohol, are depressants. It is particularly important that they not be used together. Only recently we had a fresh example of the tragic consequences when a well-known personality, under the influence of alcohol, took a sedative to induce sleep. There was no awakening, as quite often happens in such cases.

The best tranquilizer for the nervous high-strung man or woman is vigorous physical activity. I mean manual labor, such as the hobbies of woodwork or gardening, or competitive sports like tennis or handball. At the very least, a brisk walk several times a day will bring refreshment and relief. Our way of life is such that we are forced to be too inactive physically, but our emotions continue to be stimulated.

A secretary once gave me an inside view of the business consequences of unregulated use of stimulants and depressants. Her employer, the head of a small service firm, became addicted to tranquilizers. Each morning he arrived in the office in an unnaturally calm manner. He had difficulty in beginning to work, and answered his letters and prepared reports in a fumbling manner. Then he started his pep pills to see him through a business lunch. And when he returned in the afternoon, he was now supercharged. He would completely redo his morning's work, often staying until seven o'clock. This seesaw kind of operation began to have a wearing effect on the entire firm, with a consequent drop in efficiency and morale. Eventually the man had to undergo considerable medical treatment to uncover the basic emotional causes which he had been trying to cover up through the use of pills. If he had seen a doctor, instead of treating himself, his recovery would have occurred much sooner.

A Special Note on Safety

The effects of alcohol in automobile accidents are already a national disgrace. Less well recognized is the factor of pep pills and tranquilizers. Truck drivers, in particular, early latched onto pep pills so that they could sustain longer hours at the wheel. What they didn't know is that no one can predict when the inevitable letdown occurs. In no time at all the driver, who was under the delusion that he was wide awake and alert, suddenly collapses from fatigue. Numerous unnecessary accidents have thus occurred.

The driver who uses tranquilizers is also a bad bet, just as bad as the man who has had too many drinks.

Automobile safety, then, is another special reason why pep pills and tranquilizers should be strictly controlled.

No Ordinary Self-Medication

In all civilizations self-medication for the cure of illness or relief of symptoms has been in vogue. Few people are content to wait for a return to health. With the array of medications available in the local drugstore, there is a tremendous impetus to "do something."

Fortunately, most proprietary preparations as well as the traditional family home remedies are harmless. They may not actually cure, but they do not hurt. The main hazard is that, if the illness is potentially serious, the resulting delay in obtaining precise and effective medications from the doctor could be critical.

Nevertheless, as long as people are interested in health, as long as there are so many promising ads for various so-called therapeutic products, the boom in self-medication will continue. But I wish we could get across the point that self-medication with pep pills and tranquilizers is in a class by itself. There are valid medical reasons why these two items are to be taken under doctor's orders only. Those who try to get around this are hurting only themselves.

Conclusions

•Vitamins, pep pills, and tranquilizers are high on the lists of unnecessary self-medications in which millions of Americans indulge each year.

•Spend your money freely on the wonderful variety of food available in this country, and you'll get all the vitamins you need. The money you now spend on bottled vitamins can better be applied toward an extra holiday for you and your family.

•If you feel sluggish or get colds frequently, have a physical checkup—don't try to treat yourself with extra vitamins.

•Pep pills and tranquilizers can be definitely harmful. They are supposed to be obtained by prescription only and there are ample good reasons for these precautions.

•Many crimes and accidents have been attributed to the indiscriminate use of these drugs. You can help your community in cooperating with the authorities who are seeking better controls.

•Pill taking in America is at an all-time high. Most nonprescription pill taking at best will do no good and often can be dangerous to health and life. The great majority of Americans would be better off letting well enough alone.

•On the other hand, there are a few of us who have gone too far in the opposite direction. If you are one of those stoic types who won't even take an aspirin to relieve a headache, you're missing one of the advantages of living in the twentieth century. We can be proud of the wealth of readily available effective medications and the doctors who have the knowledge of how and when to use them. Make the most of these benefits.

•We well recognize the value of modern drugs and we have no intention to be negative. But there are many dangerous aspects to excessive pill taking. This is why we have put so much emphasis on the abuses—rather than the uses—of pills.

10. How to Prevent a Heart Attack

The onward surge of deaths from heart attacks—particularly in men in the prime of life—is frightening to all of us. It is ironic that medical science, which has done so much in this century to stamp out disease and lengthen life, seems helpless before this killer. Or is it?

If you're talking about a cure for coronary heart disease, such as an antibiotic, then there is little that medicine can offer. But, in the prevention of heart attacks, the answer is definitely encouraging. And the advantage of the prevention route is that it is simple—inexpensive—does not involve elaborate treatment or costly hospital bills.

In this chapter we shall attempt three things:

—to give you the information you need to help you prevent a heart attack.

—describe the ten major factors in heart attacks and what to do about them.

—dispel a certain amount of the nonsense that has been written about special diets, cholesterol, tension, and tranquilizers.

The Number One Killer

To start off, if you have the impression that there are more and more of your friends dying from heart attacks than in your father's time, you're absolutely right. The incidence of deaths from coronary disease is fantastically high, in fact it is the Number One killer of American men.

Of course everything changes, even the reason why people die. Back at the turn of the century three out of four people died of infectious disease, such as tuberculosis, typhoid fever, diphtheria. At that time, life expectancy was only forty-eight years. Since then we have gone a long way in increasing our stay in this world. At the present time any child born in America can expect to live beyond seventy years. This remarkable improvement was the result of prevention of disease—not the curing of it. And this is why we emphasize prevention.

Medical science has cut down the high mortality from infectious disease by working in the laboratory for vaccines that would overcome the virulence of bacteria and viruses that entered through the nose and throat and by way of the mouth in the food one ate. But coronary heart disease is different: it is a breakdown of an internal organ, and the preventive measures cannot be found in a laboratory.

While coronary disease has been known for over a hundred years, it has come into real prominence in only the last thirty years. In fact, until 1930, the number of deaths from coronary heart disease were so few that no record was kept. In 1930, 7.9 people died from this disease out of every hundred thousand living persons. By 1960 this had increased to 160 deaths per hundred thousand, an increase of 2000 per cent!

Why this tremendous upsurge in coronary disease in the last thirty years? There are a few obvious explanations. First, people are living longer today and consequently there will be a higher incidence of those diseases that occur later in life. If a person dies from tuberculosis at age thirty, he obviously cannot die of a coronary at age fifty. Yet aging population is a small part of the answer. In 1900, 29 per cent of the population of this country was over forty years of age. In 1960, 35.8 per cent were over forty years. This is an increase of 16 per cent, which can account for only a fraction of the 2000-per-cent increase in deaths from coronary heart disease.

It can be argued that many people who died of coronary disease in the early part of the century were not diagnosed or inaccurately diagnosed. At that time many deaths were attributed to "acute indigestion," which undoubtedly was coronary heart disease. So, with better diagnoses we would expect to find coronary heart disease looming higher. But consider this. We also have better diagnostic facilities for cancer, and are much more mindful of it. Yet cancer deaths have increased just 50 per cent in the same thirty-year period when heart disease increased 2000 per cent. There seems little question then, that coronary heart disease is the current Number One killer—and that it is on the increase.

How can we stop this rapidly rising mortality from heart disease? We do not know the cause and there is no known cure for the disease. As I said earlier there is no vaccine, there is no medication, nor does it appear that there ever will be. The only hope is to prevent it—and we now know some preventive steps that work.

First, a brief description of coronary heart disease. (Coronary refers to the blood vessels that supply the heart tissues.)

It is a very slow progressive narrowing of the coronary arteries brought about by deposition of fatty material on the walls of the arteries. It usually takes a great many years to accumulate to such a degree that it will interfere with a free flow of blood through the arteries. As the thickening of the wall progresses, the vessels finally close off. This is called a coronary occlusion, and this is what is popularly referred to as "heart attack."

While we do not know the cause, we do know ten factors

that can effect, for better or worse, the development of the disease. If you know these ten factors and how to cope with them, then your chances of being a heart victim may be vastly reduced. In fact, the best that medical science can do for you is to tell you the preventive acts, which only you can carry out.

The ten factors are: heredity, age, sex, overweight, blood pressure, stress, cholesterol, sleep, smoking, and exercise.

The Three Factors You Can't Control

Three of the ten factors can't be controlled, which is all the more reason to act on the seven others. But you should at least understand these fixed factors.

HEREDITY

If your parents and grandparents lived long, this is favorable. On the other hand if heart disease runs in your family at all, you start with a disadvantage.

AGE

Once you hit forty-five, your chances of a heart attack begin to soar. The disease occasionally strikes those much younger, but it is the above-forty-five group that is most vulnerable.

SEX

The peculiar part of coronary heart disease is that four out of five people who die from it are men. Women, up to the change of life, seem singularly immune, although in their later years they begin to approach the same incidence as men. Heart disease, then, is the Number One killer of men.

Women, with a greater immunity, also have a role to play in prevention, which is discussed in the chapter "A Word to the Ladies."

The Seven Factors You Can Control

OVERWEIGHT

*O-N—overnutrition—*is the cause of overweight and it is the Number One health hazard of our time. This was discussed in detail in the opening chapter and specific advice on what you can do about it was given. If you are as little as 5 per cent over your correct weight, you are suffering from First Degree O-N and you should review our specific steps of action in the last issue.

As to O-N's relation to heart disease, simply consider the fact that heart disease deaths occur two and one half times as frequently among persons 25 per cent over normal weight than among those of the same age whose weight is normal. Significant O-N hits one in four Americans—three out of ten business executives. Correcting O-N is the very first step you should take to reduce your chances of a coronary attack.

BLOOD PRESSURE

Increased blood pressure and coronary disease are closely related. You do not need to have high blood pressure. In many cases, high blood pressure and overweight accompany each other. And when the weight is brought down, blood pressure frequently returns to normal. But even if high blood pressure persists at normal weight, your doctor can give you effective medications that can maintain the pressure at a level approaching normal.

STRESS

Popular talk has it that the main cause of heart attacks is stress. "We're all living under too much tension, too much pressure, too much stress" is a common refrain. In my opinion, this matter of stress and tension has been grossly exaggerated. No doubt excessive tension over long periods of time is harmful and may well contribute to the development of coronary heart disease. But it is not the most important factor. All of us need some pressure and tension to be productive. There is always danger in overwinding a watch, but it is the tension in the spring that makes the watch run.

You will recall that earlier we referred to a study of the tension experienced by a sample of six thousand executives—and that we found that only 13 per cent were actually under tension to such a degree that it might jeopardize their health. Eighty-seven per cent felt no excessive strain and their work was not a hazard to their health.

It's convenient to blame our jobs for our difficulties. But in all honesty we must conclude that what a man does between 5 P.M. and 9 A.M. is more of a health hazard than what he does between 9 A.M. and 5 P.M.

So, except for very unusual circumstances, I would say to the executive, discard those tranquilizers. A little stress and pressure never hurt anyone.

Traditionally coronary heart disease has been inaccurately identified with job responsibility, typically the executive disease. Actually there is a higher incidence of coronary disease among the lower echelons of business people. Clerks are more vulnerable than vice-presidents. In a recent statistical report published by the Metropolitan Life Insurance Company (June 1967) they noted a significantly higher coronary mortality among their industrial (lower income) policyholders. This was particularly evident in the younger age groups of men, thirty-five to forty-five years.

There may be a coronary prone personality that cuts across all economic groups. It has been noted that men who are intensely ambitious, who have unusual competitive drive, and who are ever mindful of a time urgency may be especially susceptible to the early development of coronary heart disease. It could be that some correlation exists between this compulsive behavior and excessive cigarette smoking, overeating, too little sleep, and too little exercise.

Herdsmen, whose work is singularly free from stress, have an extraordinarily low incidence of coronary disease even though their diet is very high in animal fat, consisting primarily of milk and dairy products.

Even though moderate pressure and tension in our routine of living are healthful and add zest to life, those who are endowed with a personality that fosters compulsive activity may be particularly vulnerable and should try to cultivate a philosophy of a less hurried routine, including frequent short vacations.

CHOLESTEROL

If there is a successor to stress in the popular mind as the villain in heart disease, it is cholesterol. We have been inundated with information about cholesterol, yet most people can't pronounce it, spell it, or define it. So here is a very brief explanation that may dispel some of the confusion that is shared by both doctors and laymen.

First, cholesterol is not a poison. It is a very essential constituent of practically all the organs of our body, and we can't live without it. Why, then, all the fuss?

There are two reasons. First, it has been noted that the fatty material that clogs the linings of the coronary arteries is primarily cholesterol. And it has been noted that those men who have an usually high blood cholesterol level have a significantly higher incidence of coronary heart disease.

It is unfortunate that the word cholesterol has captured the popular imagination to the degree that it has. Today it is dominating the eating habits as well as the conversation of too many people. There is no predictable relationship between the intake of saturated fats in the diet and cholesterol in the blood.

Normal cholesterol values are generally placed between 150 and 260 milligrams per liter of blood. In a recent study of fifteen thousand health examinations completed in the New York office of the

Life Extension Institute the average cholesterol level of middle-aged men was 230 milligrams. When the blood cholesterol level is within the normal range, experience has shown that the restriction of saturated fat will not significantly reduce this already normal blood cholesterol, nor do we believe it will prevent the development of coronary heart disease.

When the blood cholesterol level remains persistently high (over 260 milligrams per liter of blood), it is abnormal and there is a statistically significant relationship between this and the incidence of coronary heart disease. This, however, is not an invariable finding in coronary heart disease, since more than one half the victims of coronary thrombosis have normal blood cholesterol levels. As in diabetes, arterial degeneration is a common complication when excessive uncontrolled blood cholesterol is present. Coronary heart disease is frequently an end result in both conditions.

When the blood cholesterol level persists above the accepted normal values, we should make every effort to reduce it. Restriction of the saturated fat in the diet and the substitution of the poly-unsaturated variety are musts. Just as in the treatment for diabetes, when blood sugar is increased the carbohydrate in the diet is to be reduced. When the person with high cholesterol is also over-weight, reduction in the total food intake will often bring a much more impressive drop in blood cholesterol level than that which follows limitation of saturated fat alone.

Every man in middle life is a potential candidate for arterio-sclerotic heart disease. If we were to name the five most likely factors concerned with its development, blood cholesterol, in my opinion, will be listed last. Individuals prone to develop this disease are giving too little attention to those important influences which we believe speed up the arteriosclerotic process—overweight, lack of exercise, cigarette smoking, and excessive stress.

What about diet? Despite all of the learned talk about saturated fats, and polyunsaturated fats, we cannot predict that those who eat a high fat diet will have a high blood cholesterol count, nor will a normal blood cholesterol be significantly influenced by a change in diet.

All of which is to say that if you are in the small minority of men who have a high blood cholesterol, by all means follow your doctor's advice on reducing the level. But, if you do have normal blood cholesterol, as most of us do, and if your weight is normal, go ahead and eat ice cream and other dairy products and enjoy them in good conscience.

SLEEP

We have no direct evidence of the effect of sleep on the incidence of heart disease. However, we do know that in a recent study Dr. E. Cuyler Hammond, director, Statistical Research Section, American Cancer Society, found the best life expectancy among those who averaged seven to eight hours of sleep each night, and that those who had six hours or less had a significantly increased mortality.

SMOKING

We now enter a controversial and emotional area. It has always been our policy not to deny a person anything he enjoys unless we had good reason for doing so. We have felt that the pleasure a person derives from any activity can justify assuming a certain risk. Everything we do in life for fun involves some risk. And that used to be our feeling about cigarette smoking.

We recognize that smoking has always posed some hazard to health and caused unpleasant symptoms such as the morning cough, sinusitis, chest pains, sleeplessness, fatigue, indigestion, and many others. But we always felt that, if a person thought the pleasure he derived from smoking balanced off these discomforts, that was his business. Our thinking has changed completely, and this was so before the 1964 report of the U. S. Public Health Service.

If we look at the matter only from the point of view of coronary heart disease, the evidence suggests smoking cigarettes as a very major hazard. In a study by Dr. Hammond, he found that, for every 100 nonsmokers who die of coronary disease, 210 cigarette smokers (a pack a day, plus) die of heart disease. In the recent updating of his American Cancer Society report the figure has now risen to 215 smokers for every 100 nonsmokers.

While there are undoubtedly other factors that we know nothing about, these statistics show clearly that there is a definite correlation between cigarette smoking and coronary heart attacks. (See the chapter on "The Smoking Dilemma.")

And so, if you are interested in lessening your chances of a heart attack, we have no choice but to urge that you not smoke cigarettes.

EXERCISE

Our final factor in prevention is exercise, and in my opinion this is the most important factor of all. It is so important, in fact, that the following chapter is devoted to it.

Suffice it to say here that when we talk about exercise we don't mean fifty-mile hikes, weight lifting, weekend tennis and golf. We mean walking, not riding, using stairs instead of escalators, and in every way moving around enough every day to maintain good circulation, muscle tone, and a general feeling of well-being.

It is pertinent to mention here a research study of the health habits of more than one million men and women; followed up annually for six years to record how many had died and how many had contracted illnesses.

Men enrolled in the study were asked, "How much exercise do you get (work or play)?" They were given the choice of checking "none," "slight," "moderate," or "heavy." Death rates were far higher for men who checked "none" than for men who checked "slight," "moderate," or "heavy." This was found in both the first and the second periods of the study. Among those who said that they get exercise, the death rates tended to decrease somewhat with increasing amounts of exercise.

Conclusions

•There's the story. There are ten major factors in heart attacks: heredity, age, sex, overweight, blood pressure, stress, cholesterol, sleep, smoking, and exercise. Even though heredity, age, and your sex may be against you, there are still many positive factors in your favor. Apply the easy-to-follow suggestions we have offered and the odds against your becoming a victim of a coronary heart attack will begin to improve immediately.

•Your only other choice is to become an African bushman who is not plagued by what appears to be a curse of civilization. But we think you'll enjoy life in modern America better than the African bush.

•One word of caution. We have given these suggestions on the assumption that you are in reasonably good health. Your very first step should be (and it should be repeated annually) a thorough physical examination to make sure you have no ailments that require medical or surgical correction. But once the physical examination has assured you of a normal condition, prevention of a heart attack is strictly up to you.

11. What You Should Know about Exercise and Your Heart

The present philosophy of why walk when you can ride, why stand when you can sit, why sit when you can lie down has got to go.

As one humorist said recently, even though your job requires that you sit at a desk, it's good to have strength enough to get up from the desk when it's time to go home. There may be social reasons for children riding in buses to school, but for a healthy adulthood they'd be better off walking.

But, general health aside, the main point I want to make about exercise is that, in my opinion, it is a very important factor in preventing a heart attack.

This chapter, then, is addressed primarily to the over-forty male, who is the most coronary prone in our population. As already noted, the peculiar part of coronary heart disease is that four out of five people felled by it are men—most of them in the prime of life, forty-five to sixty. And the statistics are frightening.

President Johnson, like Presidents Eisenhower and Kennedy before him, is right in his concern for the physical fitness of our citizens. In economic terms alone, the loss of life among our middle-aged men is a critical national problem. The country and its citizens have made investments in these men, have educated and trained them for complex jobs. They have now achieved sufficient experience in their businesses or professions to perform effectively. They are raising the future generation. The national benefit which we have every right to expect goes out the window when this very expensive product, the middle-aged American man, deteriorates prematurely.

We don't know the cause of heart attacks, we don't know the cure. The only hope is to prevent. In the last chapter we discussed the ten factors involved in heart attacks.

Exercise, we said, was so important that we were going to devote an entire chapter to it.

Exercise—or the lack thereof—is one condition of modern life that must be dealt with aggressively so that heart attacks among men in the prime of life may be lessened. The heart is meant to be used, our circulatory system is designed for circulation. Only some form of regular exercise can keep the human body functioning properly and can help arrest the degenerative condition that coronary heart disease represents.

What Exercise Does

Life itself is movement. The need to exercise is built into us as babies, and children do not have to be told to run, skip, and jump. But, under the confinements of the ways by which we make our livings, and with the miracle of the automobile and other forms of transportation, the middle-aged man takes the easy route. It is particularly distressing that the best-educated of us are often the most remiss. People who understand the need for proper diet, sleep, and relaxation somehow refuse to grasp the significance of exercise.

They should be reminded that the body is a balanced organism. We need food to live, but too much food is bad. We need water, but there's a limit to what we can consume. We need sleep, rest, relaxation, yet again there's a limit. And we need a certain amount of exercise each day.

Once there was a theory that a long period of bed rest was necessary after an operation. Now we know that the sooner we get a patient on his feet and walk him, the faster he gets his strength back. Moderate graduated exercise is now the treatment prescribed for convalescing heart attack patients. But why have a heart attack to find this out?

A certain amount of regular exercise, then, is vital to good health and may be helpful in preventing heart attacks.

Even the astronauts, who perform their duties by lying down, must exercise to maintain a prime physical condition.

The Link Between Heart Attacks and Exercise

I mentioned that in the thirty years between 1930 and 1960 deaths from coronary heart disease increased 2000 per cent. It was during this same thirty years that Americans started to drive rather than walk—that suburban communities were laid out without sidewalks—that a man walking down the street became a subject of investigation by the police—that the exercise in golf was extracted by the invention of the electric golf cart. Even in Atlantic City the roller chairs are now electrically powered, so the pushers can ride. Thus they will soon be in as poor shape as their passengers.

All of this may sound like a crotchety preachment against progress. It is not meant to be. I welcome every new invention, just as we at Life Extension applaud all new mechanical devices in our laboratories which make health examinations more accurate and save time. But, on this matter of riding everywhere, we have swung too far.

We forget that the heart thrives on work. It pumps to circulate the blood. If the blood has difficulty in moving, as in coronary heart disease, new blood vessels will push through (collateral circulation) to keep the muscles supplied with blood. As in a stream that is partially blocked the water will force its way around the obstruction and ultimately join up again with the main stream. Keeping the circulatory system in shape by regular exercise can help prevent blockage of the arteries.

There was a dramatic case of a laborer who died of an accident in his sixties. An autopsy revealed that earlier in his life the main coronary artery of his heart was blocked. But because he was always a vigorous man, collateral circulation was developed to supply the heart muscle with blood. Without exercise, he would probably have been dead before fifty.

Who Needs Exercise?

The kind of person we are thinking of primarily is numbered in the millions. This man is in his forties, approaching the critical age of coronary heart disease. Typically, his routine is something like this.

Every morning he steps into a conveyance, his car, his cab, limousine, or bus and drives or rides as close to his office, shop, or field as possible. (Farmers don't walk these days either.)

At noon, depending upon his economic status, he eats a sandwich in his shop, his office or goes to the executive dining room, which he reaches by elevator. If he has to go out in the daytime, he drives or takes a cab. And he returns home the same way he came.

During the day, he is subjected to all of the emotional demands of present day living, but he does nothing to work them off. At night, he increases his emotional tension by facing family problems, watching violence on TV, or reading an editorial that upsets him.

On the weekends he may play golf or tennis and he limps in on Monday morning with aching muscles and weariness.

This is the same type who, under duress, shovels snow (to get to his car, of course), has a heart attack, and reinforces the impression that snow shoveling is the cause of heart attacks. It isn't, of course. Nevertheless a violent strain on a middle-aged heart that is suddenly surprised at an unexpected call for action can be harmful.

What Kind of Exercise?

A famous educator said years ago that when he felt a desire to exercise he would lie down until it passed away. Few remember that his statement was made as a flip argument against overemphasis on college football. In fact, the educator himself kept in shape by regular walks over the extensive campus of his university.

In this book we are not talking about athletics. We are not talking about recreational sports. We are not talking about muscle building. We are only talking about the minimal exercise needs of adults.

What kind of exercise is best—the new popular isometrics, gym work, the Royal Canadian calisthenics, judo, golf, swimming, bicycling?

It is typical of our age that we seek "magic" answers to our basic problems. Hence there has been great enthusiasm for physical fitness—all right in itself—but in seeking different answers we have overlooked the simplest answer which nature has provided us. You don't need special equipment and it doesn't cost a cent.

It is walking.

How Can You Fit Walking into Your Daily Routine?

Many men who come to us say that all of this is well and good, but how in the world in our complicated society can they find the time for even walking? These same people have managed to fit in three meals a day, a bath, a brushing of the teeth. Yet they are genuinely puzzled.

The answer is relatively simple. If you leave your transportation twenty minutes from your office or shop, you will have a twenty-minute walk in the morning and twenty minutes at night. And if you pick a restaurant ten minutes away from your office, you will have a twenty-minute walk at noon. This is only one hour a day, conveniently distributed, and it should be possible for at least 90 per cent of adults. This amount of walking will work wonders for your health and may help to ward off a heart attack.

What about Other Forms of Exercise?

What we are prescribing in the hour-a-day walking routine is a minimum, of course. But it is a minimum that is observed by only a fraction of our population. What about the other forms of exercise we hear so much about? Here is a quick rundown:

Isometrics

Proponents of this widely advertised technique sometimes convey the impression that in two or three minutes you can get all the exercise you need. This is nonsense. What is isometrics? It is simply a use of the principle that if you apply pressure to a muscle, by pushing or pulling, that the muscle will keep in shape, in fact will get stronger. This is true. There is nothing wrong in keeping your muscles in shape, and there can be benefits in keeping the physique in pleasing proportion. But isometrics alone will not give you the exercise you need, because it does not significantly increase the work of the heart and the circulatory system.

The primary purpose of exercise is not to develop muscles. This is a by-product. The objective of exercise is to stimulate the heart and circulatory system and to flush out the arteries.

If you take your hour's walk, use isometric devices if you like. But do not use isometrics as a substitute for exercise.

Gym Work

This, too, is a form of body cultivation. If by gym work you mean exercises that keep the body in trim shape, this is all right. But weight lifting and devices to build big muscles are not necessary for the twentieth century. The need for big muscles has gone the way of the draft horse.

Again, if you enjoy gym work, go ahead, but don't do it in place of your hour's walk.

Calisthenics

The physical fitness enthusiasts have made a best-seller of a little book on the Royal Canadian Air Force calisthenics. These exercises are fine—particularly if you go through the routine seven days each week, fifty-two weeks each year for life. But we are addressing our remarks to the desk bound. So again we say, a little calisthenics never hurt anyone, but it is the rare person who has the patience to do them daily year after year. If you are not that person, walking is the answer.

Golf, Swimming

We are certainly for sports, particularly golf and swimming, that are sports for life. If you have the time to participate regularly, keep it up. For most people, only the weekend is available. Better do your hour-a-day walk, and you will enjoy your sports more, too.

Judo

Judo is a healthful exercise—a practical discipline in these days of street muggings and robberies—and is bound to keep one supple. But few people can indulge in it every day. Like other sports, it should supplement a walking program, not substitute for it.

Mechanical Devices

Indoor bicycles and the like have their merits. In fact, managements would be wise to provide such devices for their executives for an occasional bit of healthful exercise during the day.

The important consideration is that the exercise device chosen forces the body to work so that the circulation is stimulated. If the machine does all the work, you'll still have to walk regularly to efficiently maintain the heart and the circulatory system.

Bicycling—Second Best

A good daily exercise is bicycling. It is second best to walking mainly because it is not readily accessible to the average person. Bicycling is not only a convenient way to stimulate the circulation, but it strengthens the legs and the back and has a slimming effect.

As America builds its great interstate road system, there should be some room left to provide for cycling paths and our new communities should make such provisions also. But, until cycling is made safe and convenient, walking is our best bet.

A Word about Shoes

The lack of walking among Americans has also produced a race of footsore people. Many people, when they start to walk again, find that their feet "kill them" and they become discouraged. Much of this can be overcome by making sure you get a well-fitting shoe, and that you have more than one pair, so that the shoes can be changed daily. Apparently many men who can afford more than one pair of shoes own only one. This is false economy. The cost of a good pair of shoes is far less than visits to the doctor.

Walking and Old Age—a Bonus

A simple way to help you live to a proper age is to walk your way there. You may improve your chances of getting through the critical heart attack years, and when you get to retirement age, you will have found an extra bonus. You will enjoy your retirement much more. Today, and increasingly in the future, retired people have the means and the desire to travel. Nothing is sadder in old age than a person with the funds to travel who is chair-bound because he literally can't walk more than a few yards. So, if you aspire to tour the historic spots of Europe, wander along the Champs Élysées in your well-earned retirement, better start walking now!

Conclusions

•If your heart is now in good condition (and the simple way to find out is through a health examination)—if you are not over-weight—if you are prudent about smoking cigarettes—AND if you walk an hour a day, you have a good chance to prevent a heart attack.

•If you are a man between forty-five and sixty, you are particularly vulnerable to coronary heart disease—a degenerative condition reflecting our sedentary modern life.

•Getting back on your feet—following the simple hour-a-day walking routine we have discussed (twenty minutes in the morning, noon, and evening)—will lengthen the odds that you will beat this killer of middle-aged men.

•If you are a woman, your chances are already better because four out of five people who die from coronary heart disease are men. However, once past middle age you become increasingly vulnerable. Our advice to the ladies also, then, is to get out and walk. (It's good for the figure, too.) And you can help ward off widowhood by urging your husband to join you.

•In summation, we can answer the question—why exercise?—in two words: TO LIVE.

12. The Smoking Dilemma

(This chapter is dedicated to the seventy million smokers of America. It is designed to bring to them, in succinct form, the latest facts about smoking.)

The reports by the U. S. Public Health Service have posed a dilemma for millions of American smokers who ask, Is it really necessary to give up smoking?

Old habits die hard, and smoking is one of the most difficult for people to stop. In fact, the Surgeon General of the U. S. Public Health Service has estimated that it will take ten years to make any substantial change in the smoking rate. This is why he is concentrating many of his efforts on preventing young people from acquiring the habit.

But our question is primarily about today's smoker who says, "If I have been enjoying smoking and haven't any particular ill effects, why should I quit?"

This is a reasonable question. Normally our answer would be that anything that gives pleasure is worth continuing, within reason. We always stress moderation and balance, which is the way for achieving maximum efficiency in the human organism. Enough sleep, but not excessive—enough nourishment, but not so as to cause overweight—relaxation, such as a drink at night if you like, but not martinis for lunch.

Up until recently this has been our recommendation about smoking. Physiologically, it does no one any positive good, but we have felt that the pleasure that some people derive from it would offset any minor ailments that smoking might produce.

The U. S. Public Health report, *Smoking and Health,* issued in 1964, changed all that. To many of us in the medical profession, this was another Pearl Harbor. It is now past the time to question whether cigarette smoking is harmful. Too much evidence has been accumulated to think otherwise. The only question now is, if you are a smoker, what are you doing about it?

The Doctor's Dilemma

In more than twenty-five years of counseling numerous men and women I have learned that most people, when confronted with the realities, learn quickly to accept and to adjust their routines. A man with an ulcer understands why he must be more prudent about his diet. Someone with a high blood cholesterol will change the fat content in his meals without too much trauma.

But with smokers, it's quite different. They just don't want to accept the realities, and the resistance is formidable. In this chapter, then, we shall cover these points:

1. Review the up-to-date findings on smoking.
2. Discuss the physiological effects of smoking.
3. Offer some suggestions for smokers who wish to quit.

What Is the Case Against Smoking?

We have long known that smoking never did anyone any good physically. Now the Surgeon General's reports make it abundantly clear that smoking is definitely harmful.

Do you know, for instance, what are the two biggest killers of Americans? Heart disease and cancer, you'll probably reply, and you're right. And it is primarily in these two cases where we find a definite link with cigarette smoking.

Think of it. Cancer of the lung occurs eight times more often in a person who smokes a pack of cigarettes a day than in the non-smoker. For those who smoke between one and two packs, cancer occurs eighteen times as often. For those who smoke over two packs each day, cancer of the lung increases to twenty-one times as often as for the nonsmoker.

Of course you can point to men eighty to ninety years of age who have smoked all their lives yet are in quite good health. But remember, only a small percentage of people live that long. The rest are dead—many from cancer of the lung, more from coronary heart disease.

Authorities agree that there is probably an inherent predisposition to cancer of the lung in some people, and in this group cancer occurs almost exclusively in those who smoke. Cancer of the lung is most frequently seen between the ages of fifty and sixty at a time when there is still a fifteen- to twenty-year life expectancy. Is the fun of smoking worth risking a chance of cancer of the lung and losing out on fifteen years of life?

If you are among those who can enjoy cigarettes without paying the horrible price of cancer, then consider your heart.

Coronary heart disease is found 50 per cent more often in men who smoke than in nonsmokers.

What do these percentages mean in actual figures?

In 1962 there were 500,000 deaths from heart disease.

There were 41,000 deaths from lung cancer.

There were 15,000 deaths from bronchitis and emphysema.

The death rate for cigarettes smokers was 70 per cent higher from coronary heart disease, 500 per cent higher from bronchitis and emphysema, and 1000 per cent higher from lung cancer.

These statistics—particularly from lung cancer—are a striking indictment of cigarettes. And the same is true when we examine the over-all death rates of smokers and nonsmokers.

According to *Smoking and Health*, the death rate of those smoking fewer than ten cigarettes was 40 per cent higher than for nonsmokers.

For those smoking ten to nineteen cigarettes it was 70 per cent higher; twenty to thirty-nine cigarettes, 90 per cent higher; and forty or more cigarettes, 120 per cent higher.

Cigarette smoking, the report concludes, is causally related to lung cancer in men: the magnitude of the effect of cigarette smoking far outweighs all other factors. The data for women, though less extensive, point in the same direction.

Small wonder, then, that the prudent group of scientists composing the advisory committee to the Surgeon General put this statement in boldface in its report:

CIGARETTE SMOKING IS A HEALTH HAZARD OF SUFFICIENT IMPORTANCE IN THE UNITED STATES TO WARRANT APPROPRIATE REMEDIAL ACTION.

What Does Smoking Do?

It is true that the evidence against smoking—formidable as it is—does not as yet include exact information as to just how smoking induces lung cancer and heart disease. Some people have therefore decided that the evidence is only statistical and therefore not conclusive.

However, there are some definite physiological facts that we know.

Smoking cigarettes causes in most persons an increase in the heart rate of fifteen to twenty-five heartbeats a minute, a rise in blood pressure, and an increase in cardiac output. None of these effects are healthful.

Just what smoking does to produce lung cancer we can't say for sure. Many authorities believe that there is a carcinogen (cancer-producing substance) in cigarette smoke, and much research is being done to isolate and identify it.

Note that all along we have been talking about cigarette smoking and not pipe and cigar smoking. While the latter also have an effect, it is minimal compared with cigarette smoking. And the reason seems to be inhalation.

Cigarette smokers get their "kick" from inhaling the smoke into the lungs. Thus there is ample opportunity for any carcinogens to do their work. We have noted earlier that lung cancer develops most in those who have smoked the most and the longest time. This suggests to me that the smoke itself is an irritant and constant irritation can be permanently damaging.

We all know what happens when smoke gets in your eyes, and any fireman can tell you about the lethal effects of smoke in the lungs. The cigarette smoker should realize that the smoke he puffs from his mouth or nose has just been in his lungs, and has polluted the air from which his lungs must extract oxygen. The smoker should know that with each inhalation his lungs are bathed in dense smoke, and the breathing surface of the lungs has been exposed to it. Each time a pack of cigarettes has been consumed, the lungs have been immersed in this dense smoke two hundred times (ten puffs to the cigarette).

This is the reason, I believe, that filters have not been effective. Because the smoke itself can be damaging, the only filter that can remove all danger of lung cancer is one that will filter out all of the smoke. This is why I take a dim view of suggestions that the federal government expend money to find a "safe" cigarette. Such funds could be more usefully spent in reducing other sources of smoke such as that in our cities which further pollute the air we breathe.

But the biggest cause of "air pollution," I maintain, is cigarette smoking.

Is There Anything Beneficial about Cigarette Smoking?

The Surgeon General's committee was hard put to find anything positive to say about cigarette smoking as benefiting people—and certainly nothing that outweighs the health hazards.

In the words of the report, "The habitual use of tobacco is related primarily to psychological and social drives, reinforced and perpetuated by the pharmacological actions of nicotine on the central nervous system, the latter being interpreted subjectively either as stimulant or tranquilizing dependent upon the individual response. Nicotine-free tobacco or other plant materials do not satisfy the needs of those who acquire the tobacco habit."

This simply means that smoking is a pleasurable experience for most people which either soothes or gives a slight lift. But it becomes a habit and people who want to stop or cut down find themselves trapped in this habit. This is why more and more people say, "I wish I'd never started." They are past the point of enjoyment and are enslaved in a habit.

Some veteran smokers of thirty years or more have asked if we really believed they would benefit by discontinuance of cigarette smoking after such a long exposure. The answer is emphatically yes. Of course we realize that the danger incurred is directly related to the number of cigarettes consumed during the person's lifetime. Nevertheless it is never too late for the human body to benefit by eliminating exposure to harmful agents.

Smoking and Life Expectancy

In 1967, three years after the Surgeon General's report, there was a major conference on smoking held in New York. Much of the attention of the conferees focused on a research study that showed that cigarette smoking cuts life expectancy by as much as eight years.

The data came from a five-year study of 477,196 U.S. males conducted by Dr. Hammond of the American Cancer Society, and the startling conclusion was that the estimated life expectancy for an American man at age twenty-five is 73.6 years if he never smokes regularly and 65.3 years if he regularly smokes forty cigarettes or more a day.

Putting it another way, Dr. Hammond said that 77.7 per cent of twenty-five-year-old nonsmokers could expect to reach age sixty-five but only 54 per cent of the heavy smokers could look forward to the maximum Social Security benefits. The differences grow sharper with greater age; thus, 19.2 per cent of nonsmokers should live to age eighty-five, but only a third as many heavy smokers (6.5 per cent) should do so.

A forty-five-year-old man who smokes twenty to thirty-nine cigarettes a day should die 5.6 years sooner than a forty-five-year-old man who has never smoked regularly (and presumably never will).

All in all, said Dr. Hammond, the American male's loss of life expectancy from smoking "is not far short of the net gain from half a century of scientific and social progress." Since 1919, life expectancy for all white males has risen 4.0 years. The estimated life-shortening effect of smoking now stands at 3.4 years.

The association of respiratory disease other than lung cancer with cigarette smoking was summarized at the conference opening by Dr. C. M. Fletcher, clinical epidemiologist at the Royal Postgraduate Medical School, London, England. He said that a study of smokers and nonsmokers matched to "control most constitutional differences" had shown a "15-fold excess mortality from emphysema" among the smokers.

What if You Want to Quit?

If you have decided that cigarette smoking can cause serious disease—and if you want to quit—it's simple. Throw away the remaining cigarettes in your pocket, at home and in the office, and don't beg any or accept any from your unreconstructed friends.

Make the severance from your smoking habit abrupt and final.

This is exactly the prodecure you would follow if you were told by a doctor that you had a peptic ulcer or a coronary condition or some other serious disease that would be unfavorably affected by continued cigarette smoking. When serious illness is detected in our health examination work, it becomes our duty to outline changes in the living routine which we believe will be helpful. Often we advise the discontinuance of cigarette smoking. In such cases, we find that most men and women immediately accept and follow the recommendation.

You may recall that this was President Johnson's experience. When he had his heart attack, several years ago, doctors told him that cigarettes were "out." He took one final puff and hasn't smoked since.

You Must Be Convinced

The key is CONVICTION. When separating oneself from cigarette smoking, the psychological impact and the physical manifestation of withdrawal symptoms are in direct proportion to the smoker's conviction of the risk of serious disease if smoking is continued.

Some smokers hesitate to try to quit because of a fear that

something very unpleasant will take place. If this is your case, keep in mind that this pleasure of yours is seldom enjoyed consciously. Out of thirty cigarettes a person smokes in a day, he is likely only to really remember ten or twelve. It is true, as pointed out earlier, that nicotine does satisfy some bodily craving, but primarily smoking is habit. When the phone rings and you reach also for a cigarette, it is purely a conditioned reflex, not a bodily craving.

Many people hate to face up to going through a day without smoking. Try thinking about the periods of the day when you don't smoke, and when it doesn't bother you. Even a chain smoker doesn't smoke every minute. Every smoker goes reasonably long periods without smoking, eight hours while asleep, several hours while at the movies, in church, in a library, in many trains. While these abstinences may annoy the smoker, they don't really bother him because he is conditioned not to smoke under these circumstances.

Smoking is admittedly more than a simple habit—it has overtones of addiction. But it is not a true addiction, like a drug, where the withdrawal symptoms are real torture. Such withdrawal pains are not present when changing a habit.

Consider peanuts. Someone once defined will power as the ability to eat one peanut and stop. Many of us have learned how fast the entire bowl of peanuts can be consumed, once you have started. And, if we are counting calories, we learn to stop eating all peanuts, not just cutting down.

So it is with cigarettes. You either quit or you don't, but rarely can you cut down.

What about Antismoking Remedies?

Unfortunately there are no remedies we can prescribe that will stop the desire to smoke. Much has been written about lobeline, which is contained in many antismoking pills, but the Surgeon General's committee could find no evidence of results. This year will see many products from the "pseudopharmaceutical" industry, but save your money. These "aids" will be no more effective than reducing pills have been in effecting a loss in weight.

In spite of an intelligent realization that cigarette smoking is hazardous to health, some smokers find their attachment to cigarettes so great that separation is really difficult. They can't quite bring themselves to take the plunge. If this is your problem, we suggest a two-stage plan.

In the first stage, smoke but don't inhale. This is difficult but it can be done. During this stage the smoker can follow his usual ritual of lighting cigarettes, watch the expelling smoke, and feel that he and his constant companion are still one. The first stage must be of short duration, not more than two weeks. By this time the smoker will have found that just puffing smoke is pretty bland and does not "satisfy" at all. The number of cigarettes smoked will be considerably fewer, because when a smoker does not inhale, there is no "kick." So the transition from Stage One to Stage Two —no smoking—will not be difficult. One executive following the two-stage routine reported, "This puffing smoke in and out of your mouth isn't smoking at all, so why continue?" He was quite definite in stating that the two-stage approach helped him over the immediate hurdle.

Regardless of method, the only way you will stop smoking is to become CONVINCED that it is bad for you, and then you will find it quite easy to end the habit. Sometimes, in order to be fully convinced, people need a doctor's advice in order to persuade themselves to quit. If that is your requirement, I'll be happy to oblige, here and now.

Conclusions: My Advice to You if You Smoke

•The evidence against smoking, as documented in *Smoking and Health,* the report of the advisory committee to the Surgeon General, is overwhelming.

•As a doctor, interested in prolonging your life, I can say with authority that every cigarette you smoke threatens to terminate your life earlier than need be, and that every cigarette you smoke increases your chances of acquiring lung cancer, heart disease, bronchitis, and emphysema.

•If you are now a cigarette smoker, I can counsel you only one way: Stop. Stop calmly, unemotionally, abruptly, permanently. But STOP.

13. Understanding
Your Blood Pressure

Often when people talk about blood pressure, they speak as if it is something bad or dangerous. Actually, everyone has blood pressure and it's either normal, high, or low. Only rarely is low blood pressure reason for concern. If blood pressure is high, there is always cause for concern. Fortunately, however, modern medicine can keep high blood pressure under control in most cases.

Let's first review the nature of blood pressure and what it means to your well-being. Blood pressure is necessary to keep the blood circulating. The heart is a pump, which by expansion and contraction, forces the blood through the "pipes," or arteries. Obviously, if the pressure is high, the potential for damage to the arteries is greater and the pumping mechanism, the heart, works harder than usual with resulting wear and tear.

There is an extremely simple and accurate way to measure blood pressure. Prior to its invention by Dr. Baumann in the Twenties, measuring devices were inexact. But this device is precise and is a highly important diagnostic tool. That familiar inflatable rubber cuff which the doctor wraps around your arm is part of what is called a sphygmomanometer. The main part of the machine contains a pool of mercury in a cylinder with a glass tube attached above and a rubber connection to the cuff. It is relatively simple to determine a person's blood pressure by inflating the rubber cuff tightly around the arm, almost like a tourniquet, so that no blood can flow. Then a stethoscope is placed over one of the large arteries inside the elbow. As the pressure in the cuff is slowly released, the blood begins to flow, and a thumping sound can be heard. As soon as this sound appears, a look at the level of mercury in the machine, which now just balances the pressure of the blood in the artery, will show what is known as your systolic blood pressure. This is the level to which the blood pressure rises with each contraction of the heart muscle. As more air is released from the cuff, the column of mercury drops again and at the point where it is no longer possible to hear the thumping noise another reading of the mercury level is taken, and this is the diastolic pressure, the level to which the pressure drops between beats of the heart.

A typical blood pressure reading is recorded by the doctor as: 120/60. This is expressed as "120 over 60." The 120 is the systolic pressure and 60 is the diastolic.

Systole refers to the action of the heart when it contracts, and forces the blood from the heart into the circulatory system. Diastole is the resting period when the heart expands and receives another supply of blood.

At each heartbeat the pressure in the artery is raised to the systolic level. Between beats, it drops to the diastolic level. The pressure in the arteries is at the systolic level one-fifth of the time, and at the diastolic level four-fifths of the time. Thus, the strain on the arteries comes from the diastolic pressure to a much greater degree than the systolic pressure because the blood pressure is at the diastolic level four-fifths of the time.

What the Numbers Mean

It has been found that blood pressure varies at different times of the day and under different conditions. When we refer to a blood pressure reading, we assume it was taken under conditions of comfort and relaxation. The normal resting systolic blood pressure is considered to be between 100 and 140 millimeters of mercury. The normal diastolic blood pressure is considered to be between 50 and 90 millimeters of mercury.

There's an old rule of thumb that says normal blood systolic pressure should be "100 plus your age." This is all right until about age forty, and then it becomes too generous. The wisest thing to do is throw out this rule of thumb and find out what your doctor thinks is normal for you.

In discussing figures, we must always remember that in periods of physical exertion or emotional excitement both the systolic and diastolic pressures are raised. Such fluctuations are normal. So again it is important that blood pressure measurements be taken when you are feeling rested and calm. And if you are one of those who get nervous just because the blood pressure is being taken, the doctor may have to take it several times to make sure he gets a true reading.

Why High Blood Pressure Is Dangerous

We are concerned about high blood pressure because of the harm it can do to the heart, the kidneys, the brain, and the blood vessels in general. We know that in any pumping system the wear and tear on the pump, as well as on the pipe lines, are in direct proportion to the strain placed upon them. Let us say that a pump and pipes were made to withstand a constant strain of 50 pounds.

If the strain were reduced to twenty-five pounds they could be expected to last more than the normal length of time. On the other hand, if the strain were increased to one hundred pounds, the pump valves and joints of the various sections of pipe would soon begin to leak. Eventually, the joints of the various section of pipe soon would give way, and before long a new pumping system would be necessary.

The pumping system of the human body is affected in the same way. The pump is the heart, and the pipe lines are the arteries and veins, which comprise the circulatory system of the human body.

Regardless of whether you remember this tiny lesson in physiology or not, it is obvious that the human body is in peril if a blood vessel bursts under pressure, like a water main. High blood pressure rarely is this spectacular in its action, but the end result can be just as disastrous.

Over the years high blood pressure contributes to hardening of the arteries (arteriosclerosis). This is a gradual thickening of the walls of the arteries with a consequent hardening and loss of elasticity. Sometimes an artery will become completely blocked. The brain, the kidneys, and the heart are most vulnerable to arteriosclerotic changes. In the brain, the blood vessels become brittle. When one of them ruptures and bleeding occurs or when one becomes blocked, we say a person has had a stroke.

In the kidneys, arteriosclerosis produces a gradual destruction of normal kidney tissue with a resultant loss of function. Finally, the waste products of the body cannot be eliminated and the accumulation brings on a condition known as uremia or uremic poisoning.

But it is the heart that is most frequently and most seriously damaged by high blood pressure. There may be a hardening and narrowing of the blood vessels supplying the heart muscle with blood, diminishing the amount of blood available. Subsequently, an enlargement of the heart may take place to compensate for the extra load imposed on it. An enlarged heart is an overworked heart and consequently not normal. When the heart can no longer maintain adequate circulation, a state of heart failure exists. Heart disease is one of the major killers in this country, and high blood pressure one of the commonest contributors.

The Cause of High Blood Pressure: a Mystery

We can diagnose high blood pressure and we can treat it, but we do not know its cause. Over the years, all sorts of theories have been advanced. Salt, red meat, coffee, alcohol, tobacco all have been accused without foundation in fact.

We know that kidney disease can produce high blood pressure, but this is not common. High blood pressure also occurs in many overweight people, which is another reason for keeping your weight normal. But this is not the cause.

Others have contended that it is the tension under which civilized people live that is responsible, but this belief is not substantiated. Some scientists contend that a substance secreted by the kidneys causes the increase in blood pressure. Before we can be sure, much more research work is necessary. Some have felt that high blood pressure just comes on with advancing years, like gray hair or loss of hair. This belief is false and we do see severe high blood pressure in young to middle-aged people.

The great majority of persons suffering from high blood pressure may well inherit it. We suspect this because often there is a history of high blood pressure in parents, brothers, and sisters. The condition seems to develop without warning in adulthood.

But even though we do understand something about what high blood pressure does to the body, we don't know why it occurs in some people and not in others.

People who suffer from high blood pressure can be separated into two groups. First there are those whose pressures fluctuate from a rather high level to a normal level under different conditions. This transient high blood pressure is considered functional and probably due to nervous stimulation and therefore of less importance. The second group comprises those with true organic high blood pressure—one that is found to be abnormally high all the time.

There is no doubt that the nervous system does influence the normal blood pressure as well as the abnormal, but exactly to what extent it is difficult to determine. A physician should never be satisfied with one blood pressure reading if it is found to be elevated. Repeated observation may be necessary to determine a true reading, influenced to a minimum by the emotions. It is also important to continue to observe the blood pressure over a period of years to learn whether or not it becomes progressively higher. If it remains fixed, even at a fairly high level, this fact is encouraging and gives the patient a better outlook.

Most people who have high blood pressure never suspect it. It is detected at the time of periodic health examinations or a life insurance examination. This is one reason why everyone should have a complete physical examination by his doctor once a year.

Hypertension Is Not the Same as Excessive Tension

Earlier we discussed excessive tension and its health consequences. This condition is emotionally oriented, is usually temporary, and can be corrected when the basic irritation (job situation, family problem, etc.) is removed. It is true that under excessive emotional tension blood pressure may rise. But again, this is usually temporary.

Hypertension, which is another name for high blood pressure, is quite different. It is organic and physical in nature. Untreated, it is usually a lifetime situation.

Facts and Fallacies about Blood Pressure

Many people associate the high blood pressure person with those who are red-faced and flushed. This is not so.

Persons who are quick to anger and whose veins become distended are also thought to be high blood pressure types. Again, this is wrong. Anger will produce a temporary rise but not a permanent elevation.

Patients have come to me convinced that they had high blood pressure because their hearts pound, or their head feels "full," or they feel "full-blooded." Seldom is high blood pressure the cause.

Rarely does high blood pressure cause symptoms. Occasionally headache, commonly localized in the top of or the back of the head, is attributed to hypertension. These headaches can be very severe and incapacitating.

In fact, most people who have high blood pressure never suspect it. And since it can develop at any time, the only way to be sure is to have it checked by a doctor.

What Can You Do if You Have High Blood Pressure?

Because we do not yet know the cause of high blood pressure, medical researchers have had no choice but to try all sorts of treatments in the hope of stumbling on a cure. Some years ago, the late Dr. Herman Mosenthal, professor of medicine, Columbia University, found that one hour of rest after lunch would help to keep high blood pressure under better control. This emphasizes how important it is for the patient to have adequate rest, in fact more than the ordinary nonhypertensive person.

Another researcher, Dr. Kempner, director of the Hypertension Clinic, Duke University, learned that a diet low in salt and consisting of rice and fruit reduced blood pressure. Again, this is impractical because of the monotony and the long-term possible deficiencies in nutrition.

But research such as this has given us valuable clues in prescribing a helpful health routine for high blood pressure victims. This routine is quite different from what we recommend for the normal person.

Persons with high blood pressure should live and work at a slightly slower pace than the rest of us. They should keep relaxed, avoid fatigue. While moderate exercise like walking is always good, they must avoid competitive sports and strenuous sports like tennis, handball, and boxing.

Like the rest of us, they should keep down their weight, but this is even more important for them. There are no dietary restrictions other than the sparing use of salt.

Alcohol, if used wisely, can help to bring about a general relaxation of the body.

And, as we have said earlier, rest and sleep, the more the better, are extremely important. Ten hours in bed at night and one hour's rest lying down after lunch are a recommended schedule for people with high blood pressure.

Control by Medication

The big development in recent years is the successful treatment of high blood pressure by medication. We can now say confidently that most high blood pressure can be controlled by medications. These are drugs and should be administered by your doctor. They are easy to use, relatively inexpensive, and the treatment may add years to your life. There is no reason why, in this day and age, so many people should continue to suffer from the serious consequences of high blood pressure.

The Heart and Blood Pressure

We have pointed out earlier the damage that high blood pressure can cause the heart. Since heart disease is the single largest cause of death in this country, controlling high blood pressure takes on added significance.

A Word about Low Blood Pressure

Occasionally we hear people say that low blood pressure is as serious as high blood pressure. This is not so. Low normal blood pressure is not only not harmful, it is usually highly desirable. We do not know why people have low blood pressure unless again it is congenital, that is, inherited from a parent. We know of no adverse affects on health of so-called low blood pressure. Life insurance actuaries tell us that those who live the longest usually have low normal blood pressure. So if you feel well and normally active, no matter how low your blood pressure, you can forget about it. Just be thankful.

Conclusions

• Blood pressure is simply the force that causes the blood to circulate through the body.
• Any doctor using a sphygmomanometer can obtain an accurate measurement. The reading should be made when you are relaxed. If you are under temporary emotional tension, several readings should be made.
• High blood pressure should be corrected because it places an undue strain on the circulatory system, weakens the heart, which

must work harder, and is one of the ten major factors associated with coronary heart disease.

•High blood pressure contributes to the condition known as arteriosclerosis of the arteries.

•No one is immune from the disease of high blood pressure. You yourself cannot tell whether you are a victim. This is why it is important to have an annual physical examination, which will normally include a blood pressure reading.

•The lower the blood pressure, the less wear and tear on the heart and the circulatory system. If your blood pressure is low normally, you are a fortunate person.

•While we often say that a systolic blood pressure of 120 is "ideal," blood pressure is a highly individual matter. Only your doctor can say if your blood pressure reading is "right" for you. A normal systolic blood pressure can range from 100 to 140. Patients sometimes ask, "Which is better?" All things considered, the nearer to 100 the better.

•No one yet knows the cause of high blood pressure. But we do know that most of the time it can be controlled by medication and a change in our way of living.

•There is no reason why there are so many victims of high blood pressure. Controlling blood pressure can really be life extending.

14. The Common Cold: What's New?

Man may be ready to go to the moon, but he has yet to find a cure for the "common cold."

This universal, always annoying, and occasionally dangerous ailment is also the Number One economic health problem for industry today. Each year the common cold costs industry over five billion dollars in terms of employee absenteeism, representing 150,000,000 workdays lost.

Serious though this is to the economy, our concern with the common cold is its effect on the health and comfort of the individual. Even without a cure there are still many things that can be done to alleviate the disabling effects of a cold.

You would think that a disease that is experienced by almost every man, woman, and child would be well understood by people —at least in its treatment. This is not so. Confusion abounds—we are deluged with claims for all kinds of remedies—and many people still don't know the basic facts about a cold.

Serious research into the common cold has increased in recent years. It's generally agreed that a virus or group of viruses are the cause. But attempts to isolate these viruses or to find a way of immunization, as we have with smallpox, diphtheria, and polio have not yet been successful. So, for the time being, most of us will continue to suffer from colds. We ought to at least know how to cope with them.

Can You Avoid Colds?

Since diseases are never controlled by treating the patient, the best approach to the problem of the cold is to prevent it. The only 100 per cent way to avoid a cold would be to live alone on a desert island, because the cold germ is transmitted by people to people.

If you get in the line of the sneeze or cough or even close enough to catch the breath of someone who has a cold, you've got a good chance of catching the cold yourself. Cold germs can travel as far as six feet when a person sneezes, so it's important to stay out of the direct line of fire. Rule One, then, is to keep away from people who have colds—and when you have a cold, don't sneeze or cough or even breathe in anyone's face—and no kissing, please. Use disposable tissues rather than a handkerchief that may keep the virus alive and happy for a considerable period.

The key word about a cold is "catch." We say we "catch a cold" because we are on the receiving end. Colds are particularly contagious in the early phases, so we should avoid close contact with all members of the family. Love may make the world go round, but when you have a cold better forgo kissing your wife, sweetheart, or children.

Following this rule will help, but it obviously is not foolproof. All of us are under constant attack by cold germs. And some of us are more susceptible to catching cold than others. This suggests that there are ways to build up a defense against colds.

At this point you are going to think that I'm going to advocate eating properly, getting enough sleep, and regular exercise. And you are absolutely right. As a matter of fact, the best defense against a cold is optimum health. And good health means following certain rules.

There is no question but that people who have more than their share of colds (the average is three a year) are not in the best of health. Their diets may be deficient, they may be overly tired from lack of sleep, they ride everywhere instead of walk. I wish I could give you some magic formula instead of this "old hat" advice, but there is no magic about good health or the treatment of a cold.

How to Live with a Cold

Let's say you've done everything possible to prevent a cold, but still you notice the telltale signs—sneezing, a dryness in the nose and throat, perhaps a flushed feeling or occasional shiver. Do you have to resign yourself to suffering, or is there anything you can do?

Don't give up. You still have a chance. Cancel any evening engagements, head for home and get into bed as early as possible. Take two aspirin tablets with a glass of hot lemonade. A warm bath may be helpful, but avoid exposing yourself to drafts or cold air between the tub and the bed.

If you feel chilly, wear a sweater over your night clothes and put on wool socks. Plan to stay in bed ten hours if possible. With this procedure, you have a good chance to limit the course of the cold.

But let's assume the cold did not end with the first stage, and enters the second stage. This is when you are most miserable. One side of your nose gets stuffed up and no sooner does it clear than the other side becomes clogged. Blowing does very little good because the stuffy feeling is due to a swelling of the membranes of your nose. You may also develop a slight cough.

About now, if you are going to have any fever, you will. If your temperature rises above one hundred, it's best to call in a doctor. What do you think is "just a cold" may be influenza or, more dangerous, pneumonia. Many times pneumonia starts with the common cold. If there is nothing radically wrong, you have lost little by calling the doctor. If it is more serious, you will be in time to get effective treatment.

Otherwise, be patient, continue to get extra sleep, avoid fatigue, take aspirin, for relief of the annoying symptoms, and plenty of fluids. If your throat is sore, a hot salt water gargle may be comforting. (Use one-quarter teaspoonful of salt in a glass of warm water.) Be careful how you blow your nose. If you are too forceful, infected material may be blown into the passage connecting your ears and nose. A middle-ear infection can result.

And when you're feeling better, don't overdo for a few days. Store up some energy to enable you to resist future exposures to colds.

The Folklore of Colds: Facts and Fancies

Once I had a secretary who threatened to resign when we installed air-conditioning in the office. She was convinced that it would cause colds. Our entire medical staff could not convince her to the contrary. She was willing to have heat in the winter but not coolness in the summer.

A neighbor of mine worries every time we have a mild winter. "We need the cold weather to kill the germs," he says.

A college classmate of mine sleeps on an open porch during the winter. He worries about me in my steam-heated apartment.

I have a friend who puts on his muffler and wool hat the day after Labor Day, and another friend who goes bareheaded all winter.

All of these people have one thing in common—they are convinced that their idiosyncrasies will prevent colds.

If it makes them feel better, fine. Unfortunately, there is no evidence to support them.

Air-conditioning, if properly regulated, is one of our country's greatest boons to health. It relieves the strain on the heart from excessive heat, and it cannot produce a cold. The man who fears mild winters forgets that colds are most frequent in February and March, during the coldest weather when people's resistance is lowest and when we crowd together in transportation and public places.

As to sleeping with the windows open, let alone an outdoor porch, this is just plain foolish. When the outdoor temperature is below freezing, it would be well for you to keep the windows in your bedroom closed at night. Plenty of fresh air seeps in around the window casings. There is no health benefit to sleeping in a freezing cold bedroom.

On the other hand, certain folklore of colds has some basis in fact—at least, can't be disproved. Take the matter of chilling. Most people believe that sitting in drafts and getting the feet wet brings on a cold. Technically, all the chilling in the world can't produce a cold unless the cold germs are present. But, since cold germs are prevalent in most of the world and chilling upsets the body and lowers resistance, it is wise to keep the body comfortably warm, avoid drafts, and keep your feet dry.

The same goes for certain home remedies. Some people swear by hot lemonade; others like hot milk and honey. The common denominator is a hot drink, which is soothing to a sore throat and raw chest.

A Look at Cold Remedies

There is no medicine or pill that will cure a cold. Most remedies relieve the symptoms and make life more bearable. Most cold pills are aspirin in combination with other medications. Possibly some remedies work better for one person than another. If you find one that seems to be particularly helpful for you, use this whenever you have a cold.

However, there is no reason to take penicillin or other broad spectrum antibiotics or sulfa preparations for treatment of a cold.

All of these have their place in medical treatment, but not for colds. They should be reserved for diseases like pneumonia. If they are used too indiscriminately, you may become sensitized to the medication, and then you may not be able to take it when the antibiotic is really indicated.

Some people make a practice of badgering their doctors into giving them a shot of penicillin for a cold. The doctor, being human, sometimes finds it difficult to resist, even though he knows penicillin is of no value in the treatment of a cold. And some people are sensitive to penicillin and can get severe reactions. Let the doctor decide what is best for you. Don't tell him what you think is best for your cold.

Most of the annoying symptoms of a cold are believed to be due to an allergic reaction to the cold virus. Much of the benefit from the cold pills may result from the antihistamine they contain.

Often you have heard people say that a summer cold lasts longer than an "ordinary" cold. Such "summer" colds may actually be allergies, and they will go away only when the particular irritant— a pollen of some sort—is no longer in season. I am not talking about a recurring allergy such as hay fever which hits its victims at the same time each year. Rather I refer to milder allergies that are more frequent than many people suspect.

What about cold vaccines? Even though there is no scientific reason why they should be helpful, some people insist they have fewer colds when they take vaccines. Innumerable studies have been made and the conclusion is always the same—cold vaccines are of no value.

Influenza shots are another matter. They definitely reduce the chances of getting the flu because, unlike colds, we have identified specific virus strains. Some people insist they have fewer colds when they take flu shots. There is no reason why a "flu" immunization should affect resistance to colds, but if they do this is an added dividend. I highly recommend influenza immunization every autumn.

Some Common Questions about Colds

Over the years, I have been asked hundreds of questions about colds. Here are a few of the most frequent ones and the answers:

Q: Is it true that women catch colds more often than men?

A: Among youngsters boys have more colds than girls. When they grow older, the ladies far outdo the men when it comes to catching colds. But the reason is that they have more opportunities. Most women are surrounded by children, the group most likely to have runny noses and to be crawling with cold viruses.

Q: When do the most colds occur?

A: October is a popular month for colds. Another peak hits in January and February, and the third pops up in March.

Q: Who have the greatest number of colds, farmhands or indoor workers?

A: Farmhands. Despite being surrounded by people and cut off from fresh air and sunshine, indoor workers are less susceptible to colds than their country cousins.

Q: Can animals catch colds from humans?

A: Except for chimpanzees, members of the animal kingdom do not suffer colds.

Q: Is there any value in the saying "feed a cold and starve a fever?"

A: However it originated, this is one old saw that has no meaning. The best diet for someone with a cold or fever is a normal, well-balanced meal, in addition to plenty of liquids.

Q: Do we build an immunity to colds?

A: Maybe, but not for long.

Q: Does cold weather cause colds?

A: No. Cold weather can't cause a cold. Colds are caused by viruses, but our resistance to the virus can be lowered by exposure to cold weather. Poor nutrition and fatigue may also play a part.

Q: Why are there fewer colds during the summer months?

A: Possibly because there is less indoor contact among people— and because outdoor activity improves our general physical condition.

Q: How about age and the common cold? At what age are we most susceptible?

A: The worst age for colds seems to be between one and three years.

Q: What is the age of greatest immunity?

A: Surprisingly enough, the first few months of life, probably because of infrequent exposure to people with colds.

Q: Is it sensible to dress more warmly when suffering from a cold?

A: There is no need to wear more than you would normally.

The Outlook for a Cure

Are there any prospects for finding a vaccine for a cold which will be as effective as those for polio, smallpox, and diphtheria? I believe there are, but admittedly the laboratory results thus far have been discouraging.

It was about fifty years ago that Kruse, in Germany, published some rather slender evidence indicating that the ordinary cold is caused, not by bacteria, but by a virus. The first large scale investigation of the cause of the common cold was started by Professor A. R. Dochez and his co-workers of Columbia University in 1924. He showed conclusively that the common cold was a virus infection. However, attempts to immunize human beings were inconclusive, and all attempts to transmit the cold virus to small laboratory animals have been unsuccessful.

The outlook became more promising with a new technique of virus cultivation developed by Dr. John F. Enders, of Harvard, who, along with Dr. Thomas H. Weller, of Harvard, and Dr. Frederick Robbins, of Western Reserve, received the Nobel Prize in 1954. The Enders-Weller-Robbins tissue culture technique has opened a new vista.

One thing that has held back research has been the lack of financial support. More and more, however, as industry realizes the staggering costs of the common cold—representing 50.98 per cent of all industrial absenteeism—more money will be forthcoming. An all out systematic attack on the common cold, through our scientific resources and with adequate financing, should be successful. The unanswered question is: When?

Conclusions

•The common cold will probably be with us into the foreseeable future. On the day that science finds an effective immunization, there will be universal rejoicing—by the victims, which include all of us—and by the doctors, whose talents can better be used on the more serious ailments that plague mankind.
•But don't underestimate the seriousness of the common cold. In itself it will never be fatal, but it can weaken resistance to dangerous complications and undermine our health.
•There is no magic way of dealing with a cold. The recommended course of action is pretty much common sense. The surprising thing is that many people resist the common sense approach and cling to myths, folklore, and home remedies passed on through the generations.
•The first defense against a cold is trying to avoid it. Keep in mind that colds are caused by viruses spread by people coughing and sneezing. Here, then, are seven hints for avoiding a cold:

1. Stay out of the range of people who have colds.
2. Keep up resistance. Eat well-balanced meals and get adequate rest.

3. Have regular medical checkups that pinpoint small health problems before they become big ones.
4. If you get chilled, take a hot bath. If you get wet feet, change your socks as soon as possible.
5. If someone in your family catches a cold, move him into a separate room if possible.
6. Use disposable paper tissues instead of handkerchiefs.
7. Stay clear of objects used by people with colds: towels, telephones, and personal articles.

If you seem to be starting a cold, there are still some positive steps you can take. Here are four of them:

1. Take a hot bath and an aspirin.
2. Go to bed early, drink hot lemonade and other fluids.
3. Stay in bed at least ten hours.
4. Call the doctor if you have a temperature over one hundred. Don't go overboard with self-medications. Avoid penicillin or sulfa. Take aspirin.

•And when your cold has run its course, take it easy for a few days to build up your general health and resistance.

•The average person can count on three colds a year. This means that many people suffer even more—and many others sometimes go through an entire year without a cold. If you follow the simple rules above, you too may be one of the lucky ones.

15. Sight and Hearing

Life just isn't the same without sight and hearing. It is through our eyes and ears that we experience much of what makes living worth while. And most of the pleasurable activities of today's world —TV, the movies, the theater, radio, books—are designed to be enjoyed through seeing and hearing.

What do you need to know, then, about safeguarding these priceless assets?

First let me assure you that the outlook for preserving sight and hearing has never been better. The progress in preventing blindness and alleviating deafness has been tremendous. Unfortunately, not enough people yet understand the preventive measures available. It is estimated, for instance, that fully half of the people who lose their sight need not have done so. In other words, just by learning and practicing a few simple rules, we can reduce the incidence of blindness by 50 per cent. Surely this is well worth the small effort involved.

Here, then, is a review of the basic facts you need to know about sight and hearing.

Good Eyesight Starts at Birth

Early preventive steps can be truly effective. Back in 1908, for instance, many babies were blinded from a disease, ophthalmia neonatorum, commonly known as babies' sore eyes. By prompt attention, this disease has been reduced by 89 per cent. Only twenty years ago another disease, traced to excessive amounts of oxygen given premature babies, became a principal source of blindess in the newborn. This has been almost completely eradicated. This is why we advocate an eye examination for every infant.

But in having passed this hurdle successfully, the patient's obligation has not stopped. A child does not know how well he should see. He may have blurred vision, or see double, or use just one eye, and still not complain because he doesn't know better. Youngsters must rely on adults to assure good eyesight. By the time a child is three or four years old, his vision should have been tested. Visual defects such as crossed eyes and amblyopia ("lazy eyes") can lead to permanent loss of vision in the affected eye if not detected and treated, preferably by the age of six. Children do not outgrow crossed eyes. Eye exercises, glasses, or surgery may be required.

Eyeglasses

Prevention of blinding diseases is obviously worth while, but there are still millions of people whose vision will always be faulty because of defects in the eyeball and lens. The great savior for these people is eyeglasses, but eyeglasses must be correctly prescribed and fitted or they will be of little value. Your eyeglasses should be made just for you, so don't borrow or lend a pair of glasses or buy them "ready made" in a department store or by mail order. This sounds elementary, but it has always amazed me how many persons do not yet understand this.

Also, I'm always startled when I see someone wearing filthy glasses. I wonder how they can possibly see through them. And occasional minute spent in cleaning your glasses is a small investment of time to maintain good eyesight.

Perhaps one of the reasons some people are confused about eyeglasses is that they don't know the specialties of the various doctors in this field. Here, then, are definitions that should clarify this.

•An ophthalmologist (sometimes called an oculist) is a physician —an M.D.—who specializes in diagnosis and treatment of defects and diseases of the eye, performing surgery when necessary or prescribing other types of treatment, including glasses.

•An optician is a technician who grinds lenses according to the prescription arrived at by the opthalmologist or the oculist, fits them into frames, and adjusts the frames to the wearer. He also fits glasses to correct impaired vision but he cannot diagnose or treat eye diseases.

Contact Lenses

Contrary to what many people think, contact lenses were not devised solely to replace eyeglasses or to fool people into thinking you don't wear glasses. Rather they are better for some eye problems and, indeed, the only solution for a few. Admittedly, the corneal contact lens requires "getting used to" and some persons never feel comfortable wearing them. However, the hazards are minimal.

Safety Glasses

More than half a million Americans every year incur needless and preventable eye accidents. And if you work in a factory where the activity is hazardous to the eyes, or indulge in vigorous sports, safety glasses should be worn. Remember, there's no second chance if you lose your eyesight.

It seems obvious that safety glasses for hazardous occupations are recommended. But who is to say what is hazardous and what is not? The world is full of hazards in everyday living. Recently, for example, a man hammering a nail to hang a picture shattered his glasses with the hammer and the fragments punctured one eye.

Anyone who wears glasses while driving a car assumes a risk of serious eye injury from broken glasses. Home hobbyists who work with moving machinery are as vulnerable to the dangers of broken glasses as individuals doing similar work in a factory.

It seems only logical to me that everyone who wears glasses regularly should wear safety glasses. They are only a few grams heavier than ordinary glasses, only a few dollars more in cost, but the protection can be priceless. Accident prevention is certainly a major way to prevent eye damage and preserve sight. Wearing safety lenses of shatter-resistant glass would seem an obvious safeguard for all of us, and, in the long run, the most economical course.

Incidently, this advice is not limited just to those who now wear glasses. Do-it-yourself fans, those who operate power lawn mowers, power tools, use insecticide sprays, or students in school shops and laboratories can benefit from the protection of noncorrective safety glass lenses.

Cataracts

Cataracts are the greatest single cause of blindness among adults today. However, they can occur in any person at any age. Why they occur is still a medical mystery. They are sometimes found in a baby's eyes at birth. Some are found in persons who have worked with or have been exposed to great heat. They have also been found in persons exposed to excessive radiation or who had suffered a blow or injury to the eye. Diabetics are more vulnerable to cataracts than other people.

But most cataracts develop in the eyes of older people. These are called "senile cataracts." Senile cataracts have been increasing due to an aging population and will continue to be a major problem in the years ahead.

A cataract is the clouding of the lens within the eye that blocks the passage of the light rays needed for sight. A physical change takes place in the lens resulting in the development of small opacities. These opaque areas may increase in number and size until the lens becomes completely clouded. The eye then has the appearance of having a white pupil and is often referred to as a "ripe" cataract. At this point the patient has lost all detailed vision and can usually only distinquish between light, dark, and bright colors.

A cataract is not an infection, nor is it contagious. Furthermore, it is not a growth or, as a common misconception has it, "skin" growing over the eye.

What can be done about cataracts? Fortunately, ninety-five out of a hundred victims can have vision restored by surgery. With the advances in surgical techniques, drugs, instruments, and nursing care it is no longer necessary to wait for any particular stage in the development of a cataract. By having them removed, patients avoid unnecessary years of failing sight or loss of vision.

Although cataracts are the major cause of blindness among adults, they also hold the greatest promise for the restoration of useful vision for their victims. It has been said that there is no operation that has given so much happiness to so many people as has the removal of a cataract.

This is not to promise that the eyes will be "good as new." The surgical technique consists in removing the clouded lens, and hence the eye can no longer focus. A substitution must be made to accommodate for this before vision is restored. There are special cataract glasses that do the work formerly done by the lens inside the eye. At first these glasses may seem heavy and uncomfortable, but most patients find that this is a small price to pay for the restoration of sight and resumption of their normal day to day activities.

Recently, however, more and more persons are using contact lenses after cataract surgery. The advantage is that they provide a wider field or vision, particularly valuable in such activities as driving a car, where wide vision is a necessity. It is estimated that more than 75 per cent of the cataract patients for whom contact lenses have been prescribed learn to wear them successfully.

Glaucoma

Glaucoma is the second greatest cause of blindness in the country. There are two types of glaucoma: acute, which develops suddenly with severe pain, congestion, and reduced vision, and chronic, which attacks slowly and may occur without any symptoms noticeable to you.

The disease cannot be cured, but if detected in time it can be controlled and its progress can be arrested. Glaucoma may strike anyone, but most of its victims are persons over forty years of age. The best defense against glaucoma is a medical eye examination at least every two years, and prompt attention to any sign of eye trouble. Some of the possible danger signs include loss of side vision, blurred or foggy vision, inability to adjust eyes to darkened rooms. However, glaucoma may be developing in individuals who have none of these symptoms.

Even though you have an annual physical examination and your vision is checked by the doctor, this is not sufficient to detect glaucoma. Glaucoma is characterized by increased fluid pressure within the eyeball, which interferes with the health of the blood vessels and nerve fibers. This pressure is detectable before the disease takes full hold, but it requires a special kind of examination. Occasionally we have patients who are unfamiliar with the glaucoma examination and refuse to take it. Their fear stems from the normal human reaction that we don't like anyone "tinkering" with our eyes. Actually the examination is completely painless.

The device used is called a tonometer. First, a drop of anesthetic is administered to each eye. Then the tonometer is gently placed on the eyeball, over a sterile, disposable boot that protects the eyeball. The whole test takes less than fifteen seconds, is completely safe, and there is not the slightest discomfort. Why resist something so easy and simple that may save your sight for the rest of your life?

What about Sunglasses?

Sunglasses have only one purpose—to protect against excessive glare. Actually nature has already provided sufficient protection for most situations. Just like your fancy camera, the eye adjusts quickly to light. The "aperture" closes as more light strikes the eye, and it opens wider the darker the surroundings.

Thus there is some danger in the constant wearing of sunglasses. All of us have had the experience of sitting in a darkened theater and then going immediately out into the bright sunshine. Momentarily, we are blinded. This is the hazard of sunglasses when worn constantly. Once we remove them, the eye cannot adjust immediately and our vision is distorted. This can be particularly dangerous when driving. If you suddenly encounter a tunnel and don't remove your sunglasses you will be in almost complete darkness. It should be unnecessary to mention this, but there are still people who wear sunglasses when driving at night, as effective a method of inviting an accident as I've heard. Man survived life in the bright desert for centuries before the advent of sunglasses. Admittedly, they have a place in providing comfort under adverse conditions, but they have no place in regular use.

If you wear regular glasses, you should have your prescription ground into your sunglasses, for greater efficiency and comfort. This is particularly true if you drive a car. It is not necessary, however, to go as far as the Texan who had his prescription ground into his windshield.

Your Eyes after Forty

Thanks to the progress in surgery, medical treatment, drugs, and optical technicians the chances of a lifetime of sight are increasing for every person in the country every day. It is not necessary to accept poor vision when eyeglasses are available. It is not necessary to lose your sight from glaucoma and cataracts when skilled treatment can be had so readily.

Good eye health is closely related to general health. In a competent health examination, you will receive an eye examination and more and more doctors and clinics are adding the additional step of tonometry for glaucoma. Normally, a good annual physical examination should suffice to detect any eye abnormalities. After age forty, however, some people may find a special eye examination every two years to be necessary.

In the second half of life, numerous body changes take place. This is particularly true of the eyes. Quite apart from the disease of glaucoma and cataracts there are normal changes in the muscles of the eyes which take place in most of us after forty. Happily, glasses usually do the trick. So when you find you can read the newspaper only at arms' length, it's time to see the eye doctor. There's no need to be disturbed. It's common and just be glad that something can be done about it.

Hearing

Hearing, which most of us take for granted, is another priceless possession. Yet there are fifteen million people in the United States with hearing problems. The really unfortunate thing is that millions of them are not fully aware that they have a hearing loss.

If you have a regular physical checkup your hearing will be tested. This is the simplest procedure in the world. No matter whether the doctor uses an audiometer or more primitive methods, he can tell quickly whether your hearing is impaired and suggest what can be done.

But not everyone has a regular checkup. It is estimated that several million people right now have impaired hearing and are doing absolutely nothing about it. One research report states that the average person with a hearing loss waits five years before seeking help. This period represents a substantial loss to the person, the family, and the nation.

Perhaps more than any other physical handicap, deafness cuts you off from the world, from your family, from your friends and co-workers, and produces unhappy personality changes. Whereas most of us, in our infrequent contact with blind persons, are warmly sympathetic, we are impatient and irritated by the deaf, particularly those who are doing nothing about it.

We are annoyed by persons with impaired hearing because of certain characteristics we find unpleasant. We find these people are sometimes listless and weary, they mispronounce words, they don't pay attention, they ask for things to be repeated, they are somewhat antisocial. If the person doesn't tell us he is deaf, we write him off as some sort of eccentric and avoid him if possible. Yet if a person tells us of his handicap, we immediately try to help, because we understand.

The tragedy of it is that most deafness can be helped. If you suspect that you are losing your hearing, face up to it immediately and seek professional advice. You will save yourself a life of loneliness. The fact to remember is that if your hearing is impaired, you know it and your friends, your family, business associates know it. You cannot keep it a secret.

Causes of Deafness

Any obstruction to the passage of sound through the ear canal, middle ear, inner ear, and auditory nerve will cause hearing loss.

Common examples of obstruction to the passage of sound to the inner ear include wax, infections in the ear canal, perforations of the eardrum, infection within the middle ear and otosclerosis.

Otosclerosis is the most common cause of conduction deafness in young people, especially in women. The cause is unknown. Surgery, however, can benefit the great majority of victims of otosclerosis.

The nerve type of hearing loss is not as common. It is most frequently caused by prolonged exposure to loud noise such as that experienced by factory workers.

Other causes include infectious disease, tumors, toxic drugs, such as quinine, and unexplained loss of hearing in the later decades of life.

Care of the Ears

Keep your ears clean without using match sticks or metal objects. An occasional rinsing with hydrogen peroxide is usually sufficient. Ear pain or discharge is not normal. At the first occurrence, see your doctor. Prompt action might prevent a serious condition. Avoid swimming in uninspected pools or stagnant water. You may contract a permanently damaging infection. Avoid violent blowing of the nose or blowing one nostril while closing the other. The additional pressure can damage the eardrum.

What Can Be Done

The medical ear specialist, called an otologist, treats ears, or an otolaryngologist, who treats ears and throat, has many effective ways of treating hearing loss. Early medical treatment of ear infections can prevent permanent hearing loss. Other types of deafness lend themselves to surgery. And if these don't work, a hearing aid and lip-reading training can bring you back to a normal and happier life.

Modern Hearing Aids

Only a few years ago a hearing aid weighed a pound and a half and the wearer had to be "wired for sound." If that is how you still visualize hearing aids, you are behind the times. Today tiny transistors powered by miniature batteries make the modern hearing aid light, comfortable, and inconspicuous. Many hearing aids weigh less than an ounce, the weight of an ordinary letter. They fit in the ear, behind the ear, or are built into frames of glasses. For women, hearing aids are also built into barrettes and earrings and for men into tie clasps.

Conclusions

•Sight and hearing are a major part of living.
•Make sure that your children's eyes and ears are thoroughly checked in their early years. Teach them how to prevent accidents.
•Remember that many sight and hearing disorders, if caught in time, can be corrected by medication and surgery.
•And take full advantage of modern eyeglasses and hearing aids.

16. Controlling Cancer
What Is the Outlook?

The high death rate from cancer is no longer necessary.

Right at this moment, with the knowledge we have, one hundred thousand *additional* lives could be saved in the year ahead. You could be one of them. In fact, it is now within your own power to slash the odds that you will be a victim of cancer.

Again, as with other diseases that we have largely conquered, prevention is our best weapon. And the conquest of cancer, in particular, requires preventive action on the part of each individual.

Why do I say that one hundred thousand lives could be saved? Because great progress has been made in the treatment of cancer, by surgery and by chemical agents. But, to be effective, treatment must be started at the earliest possible moment.

You never know when a cancer has started to grow. Occasionally there are some early telltale signs, but most of the time cancer works behind the scenes. So you must depend largely upon early detection, the basis of which is an annual checkup.

We have been talking up to now as if cancer is a single disease.

Actually, it is not. It is really a class of seemingly different diseases
having many characteristics in common. Pathologists recognize
more than 150 types of malignant tumors, each having its own
specific cause. Each requires its own specific antagonist to prevent
its growth. Although the different kinds of cancer are produced by
probably hundreds of causes, they possess certain features in common. Cancer is possibly an abnormality of fundamental life processes, and remains today as mysterious as life itself.

Cancer typically begins as a "localized" disease. At the start, just
one of the tiny cells of the body (or perhaps a few cells) undergoes
an unfortunate change—it becomes a malignant cell, cancer. The
cancer cells in turn redivide and so on. All of the descendants of the
original cancer cell are themselves cancer cells. Thus the cancer
grows.

For a time the cancer cells may remain more or less together as
an intact mass, though perhaps spreading irregularly. So long as
all of the living cancer cells remain where the disease started, it is
said to be "localized."

The more dangerous phases of cancer are the later ones. Some
of the cancer cells may become detached and are carried through
the lymph channels or blood vessels to other parts of the body.
These new foci of cancer are called "metastases." But the body
has a protective mechanism. The detached cancer cells may be
trapped in a lymph node in the region of the original organ. This
retards the spread for a time. This stage of the disease is known
as "regional involvement." If left untreated the cancer cells eventually spread to many parts of the body. Death is then almost inevitable, although not necessarily quick.

In theory, all cancers can be cured when it is possible to remove
or destroy all of the cancer cells existing in the patient's body.

It can *often* be accomplished by surgery when found in the
"localized" stage, if accessible to surgery.

It can almost *never* be done once cancer cells have spread
through the patient's body.

The problem, then, is to detect cancer before it has spread so that it can be removed by surgery or destroyed by radiation.

Trends in Cancer

Dread though it is, cancer is not the biggest killer of Americans. Coronary heart disease represents 38 per cent of all deaths, while those from cancer are less than half that, 16 per cent.

Thirty years ago one out of four cancer patients survived five years or longer without evidence of disease. Now, through early detection, prevention, and medical treatment, one out of three, or 35 per cent, survives five years or more. In this sense, then, the improvements have been impressive. With our present knowledge, however, at least 50 per cent should survive.

Another encouraging trend has been the result of early discovery and treatment of cancer of the uterine cervix. Deaths from cancer of the cervix and body of the uterus have been reduced by almost 50 per cent in white women and 40 per cent in Negro women in the last twenty-five years. This improvement is undoubtedly due largely to increased use, in the last few years, of the "Pap smear," a simple test for the detection of uterine cervical cancer in an early state when the prospects for cure are best.

The survival rate for breast cancer is also improved. Moreover, a hint of the possibility of greater detection of breast cancer has been given in early results from a long-term study of an experimental X-ray examination technique called mammography. This study indicated that some cancers not detectable by palpation are revealed by X-ray examination.

In fact, the survival rate for many other types of cancer—colon and rectum, bladder—improved significantly during the twenty-year period of 1940–60.

Bucking these favorable trends are two other kinds of cancer with alarming death rates. They are leukemia and lung cancer.

Leukemia is not a growth or tumor. It is a cancer of blood-forming tissues, characterized by the abnormal production of immature white blood cells. While it strikes many more adults than children, in children the survival period is shorter. It kills about 2100 children a year. There now are some drugs that seem to be effective in prolonging the life of some victims. It is too early to feel optimistic about cure.

Lung cancer has run completely against the general cancer trend. In the past thirty years, it has increased in men tenfold and the trend is still sharply up. It is beginning to increase in women. And the five-year survival rate is a mere 5 per cent. Fifty years ago lung cancer was a rare disease. Today, among American men, it is the most common cause of death from cancer, accounting for 30 per cent of all such deaths.

Lung Cancer Can Be Prevented

We said at the beginning that cancer mortality could be slashed by as many as one hundred thousand lives a year. The major starting place would be with lung cancer, which is now producing fifty-five thousand new cases a year with only a 5-per-cent chance of survival. Fully 90 per cent of these cases could be prevented by the elimination of cigarette smoking.

The point about cigarette smoking was settled for most doctors with the report of the Advisory Committee on Smoking and Health of the Surgeon General back in 1964. We have seen nothing since to contradict the findings. In fact, they have been bolstered, for cigarette smoking has continued unabated and lung cancer has continued to increase. How in the world anyone can question the committee's statement that "Cigarette smoking is causally related to lung cancer in men" I do not know. In fact, I don't think that many people do question it, but they keep on smoking regardless.

Congress has passed the Federal Cigarette Labeling and Advertising Act, requiring manufacturers to print on cigarette packages, "Caution: Cigarette smoking may be hazardous to your health," an unprecedented step. Yet there is no halt in what the National Advisory Cancer Council calls the enormous man-made epidemic of lung cancer now extant in this country as a result of cigarette smoking.

Now it is true that a clear understanding of how smoking causes lung cancer would be of tremendous help in the development of effective means for eliminating the cause and thus preventing a large percentage of these cancers. And new information toward this objective is being obtained.

Just recently results have been published on a statistical study of 250,000 white male United States veterans that was begun in 1954 by the National Cancer Institute in co-operation with the Veterans Administration. The findings showed that cigarette smokers had a ten times higher death rate than nonsmokers for lung cancer and a significantly higher rate for almost every other disease. In one group, eleven times as many smokers as nonsmokers died of lung cancer, and twelve times as many died of emphysema, also a lung disease (and increasing at an alarming rate). The risks for cigarette smokers greatly exceed those for pipe or cigar smokers, and were lower for those who stopped smoking than for those who continued.

The relatively few who still choose to question the case against cigarette smoking point out that not all victims of lung cancers are smokers. True. About 10 per cent of all lung cancer patients have never smoked or have used tobacco only rarely. To me it is more persuasive to remember that 90 per cent of lung cancer victims are smokers. Those are still formidable odds.

Another argument is that we don't yet know the exact cause of lung cancer or what it is about smoking that brings it on. Identify the agent, they say, as you have done with smallpox, diphtheria, and other former killers, and then we'll pay attention.

I wish we could step back into history when smallpox was the scourge and ask the untold thousands of victims whether they preferred to first identify the exact organism that was killing them before accepting Dr. Jenner's vaccination. Let us never forget that vaccination against smallpox was developed long before we identified the "cause." All that Jenner proved was that his method worked and that's all that the patients of those days cared about.

Suppose I put it another way and tell you that by taking certain shots you can avoid being a victim of such dread diseases as tetanus, cholera, typhoid fever. You, along with most everyone else in civilized countries, will accept my offer gladly. Yet if I tell you, with the concurrence of most of the doctors in America and the Surgeon General of the United States that you can avoid lung cancer, you are not interested. Perhaps even as you are reading the statistics about the dangers of smoking, you are reaching for a cigarette. I don't believe that at any time in history have so many well-educated people embarked so deliberately on mass suicide. The so-called self-preservation "instinct" is indeed weak in mid-century America.

Would You Believe Early Detection and Time?

We have said that improvements in surgical techniques and new drugs have vastly increased the chances of curing or at least containing most cancers, with the conspicuous exception of lung cancer. The key—and this is how we would save the balance of the one hundred thousand lives we mentioned—is early detection plus time.

One of the reasons, for example, why cancer of the colon and rectum is claiming fewer victims each year is due to improved detection devices. The proctosigmoidoscopic examination, an instrumental examination of the rectum and lower bowel, can detect more than 75 per cent of all tumors in this region. This examination should be part of every health examination for everyone over forty.

What kind of examination is recommended in the early detection of cancer? I am often asked if there are specific tests used for cancer. Sometimes people who have had a physical examination inquire whether they were "tested for cancer."

At the present there is no single test that will indicate the presence of cancer in the body. Nor is there such a thing as a separate cancer detection examination. A physical examination by a doctor is the best single way for discovering cancer. To detect it, a doctor is dependent upon a painstaking search of the various sections of the body. In addition, X-rays, laboratory tests, and urinalysis should be included.

So when you arrange for a complete health examination on an annual basis, you are doing all that anyone can reasonably be expected to do to detect cancer.

Doesn't cancer sometimes develop very rapidly? Yes. And so if in between examinations you watch for the seven warning signals publicized by the American Cancer Society, you are protecting yourself even more. If most people did this, we would begin to see the cancer rate fall.

The seven warning signals are:

1. Unusual bleeding or discharge.
2. A lump or thickening in the breast or elsewhere.
3. Change in bowel or bladder habits.
4. A sore that does not heal.
5. Hoarseness or cough.
6. Indigestion or difficulty in swallowing.
7. Change in appearance of a wart or a mole.

If any of these lasts longer than two weeks, go to your doctor to learn if it means cancer.

Early detection, then, is important, but if no action is taken, the advantage is quickly lost. In the equation of life or death from cancer the determining factor is time. In the course of the average human life we are unmindful of time. It appears available in unlimited quantities and consequently is squandered without concern. But time becomes of the essence once a disease process begins. We all agree that immediate surgery is imperative in the treatment of acute appendicitis. Everyone recognizes the need for prompt antibiotic treatment for pneumonia. Why, then, the delay in treatment for cancer even though one suspects its presence? It is fear. The refusal to admit the possibility of the existence of cancer causes delay and time again gets its licks in.

Apathy or indifference is another ally of time. Disregarding the presence of a lump for no other reason than that the person is too busy to see about it can be disastrous. A fifty-six-year-old man, an executive, had his annual health examination, and a small, hard nontender area was noted on the side of his tongue. He was urged to have immediate attention. He explained that he was just about to leave on a month's trip and all his plans had been completed so it would be most embarrassing to change them. He was urged to cancel all plans and to have immediate treatment. Four months later he returned for examination. The tumor growth on his tongue had extended considerably. Too much time was lost, and there was now too much cancer to be cured.

Watch Out for the Quacks

Even facing up to the need for treatment is not enough for some people. They persist in going to a quack, rather than a regularly qualified physician. Today's quack trades on the knowledge that chemical treatment has improved, but he holds out hopes for cures when none are justified. So beware of unorthodox treatment, especially when medication is very expensive and payment is expected in advance. It is so very easy to check on a doctor through the local medical association that there is no reason to get in the hands of a disreputable, unethical quack.

In this day and age you would think that very few people would be fooled. Even the most intelligent sometimes get lured. I still recall the case of a learned professor of economics who became enamored of a physician who claimed to have perfected a routine of treatment that would cure both tuberculosis and cancer by diet. The professor assured me that the medical profession "would not give this doctor a chance" because they were jealous of him. This is a typical story, the usual way that quacks justify their lack of recognition.

To convince my friend that the doctor in question was a quack, I agreed to observe some of his patients. I asked that he send me six of his patients with pulmonary tuberculosis for examination. Then the doctor would treat them according to his dietary routine and return them to us when they were cured. Our examination revealed that not one of these patients had tuberculosis in the first place! Our quack had simply told them that they were tubercular and promised a cure in three months. It is indeed easy to cure a disease that never existed, and it is no wonder that such patients spread the word to their friends about their marvelous doctor.

Conclusions: What You Can Do to Prevent Cancer

It is our belief that eventually the massive research on cancer will bring us the answers we need in order to control cancer—just as we have tamed many formerly deadly diseases. But until that time, the situation is far from hopeless. Even though we don't know what causes cancer, we know many things that will prevent it or cure it. Here, in summary, are the rules you should follow:

1. DETECTION. The earlier we can detect cancer, the greater the chance of arresting its development. This means having an annual health examination—and I mean *annual*—not every few years. This examination should include a complete physical examination of the body for signs of cancer—a proctosigmoidoscopic examination, a chest X-ray, blood tests. For women the "Pap smear" is essential.

2. PROMPT ACTION. If any tumor is discovered, seek medical treatment immediately. Do not delay.

3. WARNING SIGNALS. In between your annual examinations, keep in mind the seven warning signals mentioned earlier. If you

find one, go to your doctor right away. There may be nothing wrong, but it's better to find out for sure.

4. SMOKING. If you are a cigarette smoker, stop now. At the very least, cut your smoking in half. Or switch to a pipe or cigar. Reread the section on lung cancer and smoking until you are as convinced as I am that the elimination of cigarette smoking is the single most important way to slash the casualty rate from cancer.

5. FEAR. Many people so fear cancer that when they suspect its presence they are afraid to go to the doctor. There is much more to fear in not going to the doctor. Cancer does not cure itself. Everyday we are learning new and better ways of treating it.

6. QUACKS. Avoid all so-called doctors who promise quick cures, who prescribe strange diets, or who demand payment in advance. If you are not certain about your doctor, consult your local medical society. A phone call is all you have to make to get the correct information.

17. A Word to the Ladies

Special Health Problems of Women

Since the days of Lydia Pinkham, women have been the increasing target of pharmaceutical and cosmetic advertising aimed to correct a frightening array of "diseases and disorders" supposedly unique to them. This outpouring of facts and "minifacts" suggests that we devote a chapter to special health problems of women.

Practically everything we have written in past chapters on health—exercise, heart, cancer, vitamins, drinking, eating—applies to women and men alike. Some of the products and advice aimed at women alone are just as valid—or invalid—for them. The health rules for humans are basically the same for men, women, and children.

Admittedly, however, women are different both physiologically and psychologically. The story is told that if you ask a man where he obtained the steak he is serving you for dinner, he'll give you the name of the butcher. But if you ask a woman, she'll say,

"Why? Is there something wrong with it?" This suggests that many times women by nature and the role they play in our society are "worriers." They worry about their husbands, their children, whether they are still attractive, and they worry about their health.

They are also plagued by numerous minor but uncomfortable ailments that come about because of fashion and the quest for eternal youth. Most women seem to be naturally able to endure pain better than men, but why they willingly suffer discomfort for fashion's sake is something men will never understand, nor should they try. Nor do I propose to discuss miniskirts.

Fashions, however, to which women are devoted, create various health problems, and there is little that a doctor can do about them. If the fashion is to wear tight shoes, it is probable that permanent and painful damage will be done to the feet. If the style is for a deep mahogany tan (sun-induced), there is bound to be a greater tendency toward skin cancer. I well recognize the futility in talking down such unhealthy practices, because fashion is here to stay. Fortunately, fashion changes and we can always hope. There is one current fashion, however, which I hope remains and that is the vogue for weight control. Obesity is in danger of becoming a national disease and is known to be a negative factor in longevity. So if it's the fashion among women to be slim, I'm all for it.

Some advertisers trade on the fears and apprehensions of women. It is claimed, for instance, that women until the age of fifty-five are in need of extra iron and therefore should use iron supplements. There is no basis for this generalization. The standard laboratory tests in a good health examination will reveal whether there is such a deficiency, and then it is up to the doctor to determine the cause and to prescribe.

Women, I have said, are often apprehensive about trivial matters. However, on a less frivolous level, there are two worries which most women have—about cancer and the menopause—and I will discuss them in some detail.

New Hope in the Battle Against Cancer

Cancer strikes men and women both. However, women have two special concerns, cancer of the uterus and of the breasts. Fortunately, the odds are constantly improving due to the improvement of techniques for early detection. As I mentioned, deaths from cancer of the cervix and body of the uterus have been reduced by almost 50 per cent in white women and 40 per cent in Negro women in the last twenty-five years. This encouraging development is doubtless due largely to the use of the "Pap smear," a simple test for the detection of uterine cervical cancer in an early stage.

I am convinced we could save the lives of many more women if they had this test every year, without fail, along with a full health examination. A health examination, as I've explained earlier, includes cancer detection. In addition, every woman should make sure that her doctor provides the "Pap smear."

The survival rate for breast cancer is also improved. There is now a new X-ray examination technique called mammography, which promises to give more precise results than the conventional palpation method.

Why don't more women avail themselves of these lifesaving techniques, which can also give them peace of mind? Besides the factor of fear, which most of us have, some women are deterred by feelings of modesty and possible embarrassment. In modern America, however, it is now easier to find a doctor or clinic where examinations can be in the utmost privacy and convenience. For those who prefer women doctors, there are an increasing number available, and some examination clinics offer a choice.

I stress the importance of annual examinations for women because we have proof that the cancer death rate is steadily being reduced. These two special problems of women need no longer be the peril they once were if you will take advantage of these medical tests I have described.

On the other side of the coin, women are amazingly free from lung cancer. The great preponderance of lung cancer is in men and just why we don't know. One plausible theory is that not as many women have been smoking as men, nor for as long a time. This seems substantiated by recent figures that show a slight increase in the rate of lung cancer in women. So I can only counsel you to stop smoking or, better still, don't start the habit.

For a fuller discussion of cancer as it applies to both men and women, please refer to Chapter 16.

Some Observations on the Menopause

The menopause has been a traditional worry among women since the beginning of time. In less knowledgeable periods of history, women looked up it as the end of life and, even today, I am distressed by the number of women who view it exactly the same way. We have much evidence that this does not have to be. For every woman who finds the menopause a difficult time, there are two who are not even aware that they have made the transition.

One of the genuine fears of some women is that they will become suddenly prematurely aged—their hair will turn gray overnight, their skin will become wrinkled, coarse, and hairy. Again, this does not necessarily have to happen. We cannot stop the aging process in human beings, but women can age as gracefully as men.

When we talk about premature aging, let's first recognize that this can happen in men as well as women. It is not necessarily related to the menopause but it does have to do with practicing the rules of health.

Another part of the problem of the menopause is psychological. Women by nature value their appearance, and to them the menopause triggers the thought that old age has arrived. The menopause is a time of life in our society when many women find their children have left home. There are adjustments to be made; there are some tears for the "days that are no more." There are emotional difficulties and they too are blamed on the menopause. Conversely, women with more than their share of emotional problems find these feelings intensified during the menopause.

Another myth is that the menopause means the end of sexual relations. Not only is this untrue, but many women feel relieved by the loss of their fear of pregnancy and enjoy sexual relations even more.

All of this suggests that by mental preparation many of the difficulties of the menopause can be avoided. Women who recognize that their children will grow up and leave home, and who plan in advance some substitute activity, are less likely to "menopausal depression."

For any husbands who may be listening in, let me say that you can be a big help in this advance preparation. I emphasize the word *advance*. Many popular articles on this subject advise the husband to be particularly understanding and sympathetic and kind, etc., during this difficult adjustment period for his wife. This is well and good, but from a practical point of view it is better to face up to the matter before it happens.

If a husband will share with his wife the problem of what she will do when the children leave, what their joint retirement plans are—if he will recognize that when the time comes it will require some mutual adjustment—then the chances are good that the problem won't come up in the first place. In many cases, I have noted, the menopause is a symbol more than a reality. It is a test of a marriage and, if it hasn't been a particularly good marriage, this is sometimes the excuse, rather than the reason, for its collapse.

I have emphasized the emotional and psychological aspects of the menopause because they are the predominant ones, in my experience. This does not mean, however, that there is not a physiological aspect or that there is no role for medicine. Indeed, there is a stronger role for medicine than ever before and it is an encouraging one.

Can You Remain "Feminine Forever"?

One gynecologist, in fact, is convinced that the physiological aspects of the menopause can be completely eliminated through hormone therapy. In books and articles he has promoted the notion that you can remain "feminine forever"—and one of the ads proclaims that you can learn "how to avoid menopause completely in your life, and stay a romantic, desirable, vibrant woman as long as you live." Another doctor has stated that the menopause is "one of nature's mistakes" and should be eliminated.

Since many women have doubtless read these accounts in detail, I'd like to give you my considered views on these claims. First of all, I certainly don't agree that the menopause is a mistake of nature. The statement is based on the fact that the human female is the only animal whose ovaries stop functioning some years before the normal life span ends. I don't consider that a mistake; I consider it a blessing. Unlike other animals, the young human needs maternal care for many years, not a few weeks or months. Would a seventy-five-year-old woman want to start raising a family? No, I think that the menopause, in stopping the capacity to reproduce twenty to twenty-five years before the biblical threescore and ten, is deliberate and wise.

However, if these doctors mean that with new hormones certain physiological discomforts associated with the menopause could be minimized, then I am in agreement.

First let me explain what I think may sometimes be a misunderstanding between the menopause and the cessation of the ability to reproduce. The hormones we have referred to are the sex hormones. In both men and women, the supply of these hormones contributes to our general physiological well-being, and part of aging results from a decrease of these hormones. In men the body's production of sex hormones diminishes gradually with advancing age. But when the ovaries—which are part of the reproductive apparatus—cease functioning, there is also a drop in estrogen and progesterone, the female sex hormones. It is this drop that brings on many of the symptoms we customarily associate with the menopause—forgetfulness, losing things, irritability, hot flashes, wrinkling skin, drying of the sex organs, and flabbiness.

Now it seems to be pretty well demonstrated that in many cases estrogen therapy will eliminate these symptoms.

Estrogen is also thought to be important in the formation of bone. Postmenopausal women sometimes suffer from osteoporosis, a progressive thinning out of the bones which makes them vulnerable to fractures.

There has been good reason, then, in the past, for women who have seen these effects in their mothers and aunts, to have a dread of the menopause. Fortunately, in many cases estrogen therapy will minimize these menopausal symptoms and maintain the physiological conditions. Aging will be gradual rather than abrupt.

Some doctors have hesitated to use estrogen because they feared that it could induce cancer. However, many endocrinologists and gynecologists question the evidence for this concern.

It has been our belief that caution in medical matters is the best policy. However, when a treatment emphasizes a preventive approach, I believe it warrants serious consideration. I am particularly interested in the preventive aspect of estrogen and the menopause.

"Preventing" the Menopause

The leading proponent of hormone therapy for the menopause would start treatment early in life. If tests revealed a deficiency, treatment would be given until the estrogen level was normal. In this way, it is thought, the menopause could be completely eliminated.

I would prefer to recommend a slightly different approach because I believe in treating the whole person. As we discussed earlier, there are many factors in the menopause besides the purely physiological. And there are many other preventive steps a woman can take to increase the chances for a healthy, happy, and long life. The firm establishment of the regular rules of health is the first place to start. Next, the annual health examination should become habitual, and it should include the Pap smear for cancer. At the same time, the same Pap smear will provide an evaluation of the hormone level. When estrogen deficiency appears, appropriate action can be taken, just as you would do if other laboratory tests revealed deficiences.

For those women now approaching the menopause, and having symptoms, I would certainly recommend discussing with your doctor the advisability of estrogen treatment. The results seem encouraging and the treatment safe. I would not want to promise everything that some of the ads have so blatantly proclaimed, but in general I approve.

Women's Role in Family Health

In talking to married women about health, I also like to stress a point that may seem off the subject, but it is most important, I believe. One of the normal fears that any wife has is the health of her husband. And in mid-century America this is becoming a very real fear for women whose husbands are in the critical decades of forty-five to sixty-five. This is the period when heart disease—which is much more likely in men than women—is liable to strike. It is not a pleasant prospect for a woman to contemplate becoming a widow long before retirement age.

Rather than just worrying, there are some positive things you can do. A factor in heart attacks is emotional stress. A man must have a chance to relax and recoup his nervous energy. Coming home to a warm, friendly welcome will help him do this.

You have the opportunity through the meals you serve to keep his weight within bounds. And by keeping a sensible social schedule, you can help him get enough sleep, another important factor.

Exercise is essential in preventing heart attacks. Try to encourage your husband to walk as much as possible. Walk together if you can.

Regular vacations are important and you can see to it that they provide a change of pace, a change of scene, and that they are within your budget. (The emotional stress and worry from the unbalanced family budget can be a greater hazard to health than business problems.)

Finally, make sure your husband gets a physical checkup each year. If his company does not provide it, make this part of his birthday present to you.

Sometimes when I've told women this, they say, "Look, I work too. I have plenty of troubles of my own." True. However, women seem better able to cope with a great variety of stresses than do men. The incidence of heart disease among women, as we have discussed, is not at all as serious as among men. That's why I want you to understand how important your role is in helping your husband live longer.

In our family structure, women also play an important role in health education. The reason there are many people today who still do not understand the basic rules of health is that their mothers did not teach them properly. Most of us are accustomed to lean on the mother in the family when it comes to problems of health, nutrition, and hygiene. The more that women keep up with medical developments that affect health, the better chance we'll have for a fit citizenry.

Conclusions

•The basic rules of health are much the same for women as for men. However, women have some special problem areas where preventive action is necessary and effective.

•The incidence of cancer of the uterus and the breasts is lessening due to the use of diagnostic examinations.

•Cancer deaths can be limited even more if women will have regular periodic examinations.

•The menopause need not be troublesome if the proper mental preparation is made and advantage taken of estrogen treatments when needed.

•Women have a special role in safeguarding the health of their families and in transmitting the basic rules of health.

•Women are often burdened by fears, large and small, because of their roles in our society. Kindly reassurance and understanding by men—and this includes doctors—will go a long way in helping women maintain continuing good health.

18. The Annual Examination
Foundation of
Preventive Medicine

Health examinations are the basis of preventive medicine. Periodic checkups give you a chance to get medical treatment in time, and at much less cost, than if you wait until some disorder has reached the emergency stage.

What constitutes an adequate examination? How much time should it take? How much should it cost? Where should you go for an examination? These are questions that often are asked.

What a Typically Modern Examination Should Include

A typical modern examination should include the following:
A detailed history of symptoms and habits of living.
A complete physical examination.
Laboratory investigations, including:
    a urinalysis
    examination of the blood for anemia and other blood diseases

chemical tests of the blood for sugar content to detect diabetes

uric acid content to detect gout

urea nitrogen content to detect kidney dysfunction

a cholesterol determination

an electrocardiogram, to indicate impaired coronary circulation and disclose abnormal rhythm or rate of the heart

a chest X-ray, to detect tumor growth or infection in the lungs, and also to establish the size of the heart

a gastrointestinal X-ray, to detect ulcers or tumors

for those over age forty, a proctosigmoidoscopic examination to detect tumors or other pathology in the rectum and sigmoid.

(The blood test may seem formidable, but for the examinee they require only one small sample of blood. The rest is up to the laboratory.)

When all the reports of the examination are assembled, there should be a conference with the doctor. At this point he will give a realistic evaluation of any abnormalities. He will also call attention to those habits of living that are not consistent with good health. For instance, people frequently stray from the eight hours of sleep and the twenty minutes of outdoor walking three times each day so necessary to well-being. We need to be reminded that overnutrition is malnutrition and that sometimes a more moderate routine of eating is in order. And a firm recommendation to discontinue cigarette smoking occasionally spurs a latent desire to quit into a reality.

The reassurance and peace of mind that follow the health examination when all is well easily justifies the time and expense. Or, if pathology is detected, the examination could be lifesaving.

Another reason for an annual health audit is to clear your mind about any symptoms that annoy you. All of us, as we grow older, experience various annoying discomforts—a pain in the chest, a twinge in the arm or leg—a small lump under the skin. The chances are that most of these symptoms are not indicative of any disease. The best way to deal with them is to have a checkup and find out, and then dismiss them from your mind.

What about Cancer Detection?

Many people are impressed with the importance of periodic checkups for cancer. They are right in so believing, for cancer is one of the insidious diseases to which we have referred. Thus we are often asked what is involved in a cancer detection checkup.

The answer is simple. A comprehensive health examination is a cancer detection examination.

So, a proper regular health examination is what the Cancer Society (as well as the Heart Association) recommends, so that abnormal conditions can be discovered.

Where to Get a Physical

A person need not go to the hospital for his health examination. This is sheer luxury and extravagance, as well as exhausting. There is no investigative procedure required as part of a health examination that cannot be carried out satisfactorily in a well-equipped doctor's office or a clinic. There are not enough hospital beds, and they should be reserved for sick people.

If the family doctor has adequate equipment and can devote sufficient time, he should do the examination. Some family doctors, however, are so busy caring for sick people that their time for examinations is limited.

So, the outside clinic sometimes is best. Such clinics usually refer you to your own doctor if anything wrong is detected. Some will provide treatment as well. In either case, it is wise to determine whether the clinic has a full range of specialists, fully qualified to evalute the examination findings—whether it has its own laboratory—how long it has been established. Any reputable clinic will be more than willing to answer these questions without any obligation.

Incidentally, we hear so much these days about "executive" examinations that some people believe that many clinics are limited only to businessmen. With a very few exceptions, this is not so. The clinics we have in mind serve both men and women regardless of occupation.

It is true that many business firms and trade associations have long recognized the economic value of making sure that their executives, in whom so much money has been invested, keep in good health. Many of them pay for annual physical examinations for these executives, either at private clinics or in their own medical departments. Many other progressive organizations recognize the value of extending this service to all employees, as well as providing preemployment and prepromotion examinations. After all, these same companies offer insurance benefits if one has an illness or dies. Health examinations are positive ways to prevent disability and extend life.

What about Time and Cost?

We have already said that a health examination need not be time-consuming. For those under forty a highly adequate examination can be conducted in one two-hour visit. For a very comprehensive examination, the amount of time need not exceed four hours.

The costs of these examinations are not excessive. For those under age forty, the range should be forty to sixty dollars. For a more comprehensive examination, including a gastrointestinal X-ray series, the cost should range from seventy-five to one hundred dollars. There are hospital clinics where the costs are even lower, but there one is subjected to longer waiting time than in the clinics to which we refer.

In any event, it is not necessary to pay more than one hundred dollars for a competent health examination.

It is a valuable investment in your future.

Conclusions

•Prevention is the single best way to maintaining good health, and an annual examination is the basis of preventive medicine.
•An adequate examination can be obtained nearly anywhere in the country.
•The time needed is less than four hours in most cases.
•The costs are modest—about the same as one monthly payment on a small automobile.
•Why are you waiting?

19. It's Your Attitude That Counts

A Sense of Well-Being Is the Goal

Your mental attitude is probably the single most important factor in maintaining good health through life.

I am not talking about mental illness, neuroses, or other psychiatric problems. I am referring to your outlook on life. This may seem a strange approach for a doctor to take. But as one who stresses the preventive approach, rather than waiting until something drastic has happened, I have learned that attitude is very important.

Let's examine for a moment what we mean by good health. Technically, you could say that it is the absence of disease or physical disorder. But many people who qualify in this definition do not necessarily have positive good health. By positive good health, I mean a sense of well-being.

We all know the person who drags himself to work, is morose, whines, and complains. While no disease is present in the body, you can't call this a truly healthy organism. In fact, this kind of person in an organization can have a detrimental effect on the general well-being of the others around him, which shows the destructive power of this kind of negative outlook.

There's no question but that the cheerful, optimistic person has the better of it when it comes to good health. And this positive attitude actually can ward off disease and minor illnesses—just as a dour attitude seems to bring on all kinds of nagging ailments.

And America is certainly a country of citizens with minor ailments. Just think for a moment of the medications that are heavily advertised in buses and trains, on TV, in magazines, and that obviously must have a large market. They are primarily nostrums for nervousness, tension, stomach upsets, and headaches.

A current commercial shows a woman listening to her children bang pots and pans in the kitchen. A rope, stretching tighter and tighter, symbolizes that her nerves are reaching the breaking point. And then she takes a dose of the "magic" product and is once more at peace. Now small children have always been mischievous and noisy from the beginning of time, yet most mothers have survived. They had not collapsed so abjectly.

Stomach upsets, another favorite TV subject, are much more likely with the negative type personality. This has been so well observed in the past that we find the word "dyspepsia," meaning stomach disorder, has a recognized second definition, "gloomy or irritable." So the bickering that takes place at many American dinner tables is the good ally of the stomach remedy. It is far better to create an atmosphere of cheerful surroundings, good talk, and laughter than to reach for a pill.

Headaches, unless the result of a serious illness, are a rarity with the person who has a good outlook on life.

"Volunteer" Sickness

So despite the miracle drugs, the new skills in surgery, the fantastic advances that are being made in technology for the treatment of serious diseases and accidents, the quality of American health is not of the best. The answer is not to be found in the laboratory. It is to be found in the quality of our American life.

We find ourselves allied with the ministers, editorialists, sociologists, and other observers who are deploring the apathy that is said to be so widespread throughout our country. This same apathy breeds poor health, for in such persons there is obviously no sense of well-being—only a kind of apprehension or withdrawal.

A prominent management consultant told me that the lack of a proper attitude is the biggest problem faced by employers. They heap on the benefits—more paid holidays, bonuses, pensions— yet the productivity they are after does not result. As a doctor, I know the types of persons he means. They are the ones who are overdrawn on their sick leaves, who fill the doctors' offices, who buy the pills and the headache powders. Yet there is seldom anything truly wrong with them medically. Rather you can say quite accurately that they "enjoy" poor health.

Now I do not for the moment question that these people have these headaches and upset stomachs. The disorders are real. What I am saying is that most of the time it is their attitudes toward life that have brought on these physical ailments.

Dr. Eric Berne, author of the best-selling book *Games People Play,* calls such people "losers." "Losers," he says, "spend their lives thinking about what they're going to do. Winners, on the other hand, are not afraid to savor the present. Winners are enlightened people who grow rich, healthy, happy, strong, wise, and brave using just three words in life: Yes, No, and Wow: 'Wow' is to express the healthy, childlike wonder in all of us."

Dr. Berne's "winner" sounds like my optimist who has a sense of well-being.

I have also been struck by the wisdom of the observation by C. Northcote Parkinson, who points out that "The busiest people have no time to be sick. Executives who are, or think they are, indispensable at the office have minor indispositions that begin Friday night and disappear by Monday morning Their major illnesses immediately follow the end of some major task and if the work continues at crisis level they do not fall sick at all. They become as immune as physicians during an epidemic, mothers with large families or sailors during a gale at sea."

Then he gets at the heart of what I am saying: "This known fact would convince us—even if we did not already suspect—that there is a voluntary element in many an illness. The patient has dropped his subconscious guard and allowed himself to collapse. He wants a rest and can see no other way to get it."

If there is a "volunteer" element in getting sick, there is also a will to remain healthy. There is no question but that the body has powers to resist disease. This was recognized by Hippocrates, who spoke of the body's healing powers, which are operated by the individual's own nervous vitality. The people who don't take advantage of these powers really don't want to. To these people, an ailment acts like a fuse on an overloaded wire. When too heavy a load is put on them—problems at the office or at home—a minor illness becomes the way out. A periodically slipping disc is one of the commonest, or we may take advantage of whatever epidemic happens to be available. What we catch is undoubtedly an infection, but we can't always put the blame on the germ or virus concerned. We all breathe in billions of disease agents daily, but we catch the diseases only when we need to—when, through our lowered nervous vitality, we give them permission to take over.

Part of the problem is a failure of adaptation. Primitive man, when frightened, instinctively prepared to fight or flee through a number of reflex actions. Among them, his digestive system stopped working, to concentrate his body's energies for the challenge. Like primitive man, our digestive processes stop or slow down whenever we are worried or anxious. But often we don't take the hint. We continue to eat and drink with unfortunate results for our digestions.

Experiments have shown that when a modern man undergoes a modern fear, like the threatened loss of his job, his stomach promptly records the shock. Or, if we have certain worries but can't do anything about them, we have feelings of frustration. Dr. Hans Selye, of the Institute of Experimental Medicine and Surgery,

University of Montreal, studied the physical results of frustration in his laboratory. He strapped rats to a board, a frustrating experience for them. As they struggled in vain, large patches of their heart muscle underwent acute disintegration and the animals died.

It is easy to see that the only way to save the rats would be to release them from their frustrating experience. But frustrations in modern life are not so apparent as in this laboratory experience. When we don't feel well, we demand that medical doctors treat us with drugs. They may relieve, but until the frustration is removed, they will not cure.

The ball is back in your court again. You are the only one who can figure out what it is in your particular situation that is upsetting you, producing worries and frustration. Unlike the rat in the experiment, we are not irrevocably strapped to a board. There is usually something that can be done, either to adapt to one's particular circumstance or change it. And then we can once more depend upon our natural vitality to keep us well.

Again, referring to the "volunteer" element in health, some people deliberately set out to make themselves old looking. In so doing they begin to age faster. Why do they do this? Part of the reason, I believe, is that they subscribe to myths. They associate overweight with maturity, for instance, so do not worry about keeping down their weight. Among women, this is shown by a lack of interest in new clothes. Now in my experience, it just isn't normal for a woman not to be interested in new clothes. So if a wife still changes her wardrobe completely each year, the husband should be glad that she is "with it," that she is interested in what is going on around her.

Feeling Sorry for Oneself

Another factor in "volunteer" sickness is dwelling too much on oneself. This is why major religions have taught the efficacy of contemplating a larger being, to get us to forget about ourselves.

And the person who has a mission in life, an interest in others, achieves the same effect. He forgets himself, which, within obvious limits, is one of the key steps to good health.

The negative personality, or just generally apathetic person, is aware that something is wrong with him. So he seeks relief for his dull inner ache in ways that constitute major health hazards. Feeling sorry for oneself—an amazingly prevalent phenomenon in affluent America—has led to the development of two lethal pastimes, smoking and alcoholism.

People who believe "no one cares" "pleasure" themselves with a cigarette, which they feel they've earned because of their sorry lot. "I needed that," they may say with satisfaction as they take a drink. Maybe in a sense they did, for alcohol soothes tension, but they don't need the third or the fourth drink, which cause the trouble.

Some people say that the pace of modern society—and no one will deny that twentieth-century living has its problems—is such that these palliatives are necessary to survival. But a soaring lung cancer rate and alcoholism in the epidemic stage are not to me solutions.

It seems to me that a better way to get at the problem would be to look at the other side—the number of people who don't need these crutches, who manage to get along without too much difficulty, or, in Dr. Berne's term, "the winners."

Over the years it has been my good fortune to know many successful executives in all kinds of fields. Contrary to what we are often told, the top people suffer few of these minor ailments we've been discussing. Even though their work hours may be long, they are moderate in their use of alcohol, and the majority are non-cigarette smokers. In fact, if you note the various write-ups of executives which appear in various financial magazines and on the business pages, the very normality of these people is the most striking factor. Apparently, in adjusting to their life's work, they have also learned to adjust to life in general.

There was an article in the papers recently about business luncheon clubs in New York. All of them mentioned were expensive, available only to a select number of men who can afford the best. Yet the chefs bemoaned the fact that most of the requests were for plain, light meals—fish seems to be the predominant favorite— and the bar is only lightly patronized.

Here are people who can have anything they want, and, when given the choice, they are relatively Spartan in their demands. The answer, I'm sure, is that they are so interested in what they are doing that they have no desire to go overboard on drinks or food. They prevent the stomach upsets, the nervousness, the headaches that so many others accept as a regular way of life.

To the medical profession, the frustrating feeling is that the kinds of problems we can do something about, if only a little effort is shown on the part of the patient, seem the most difficult. I have known handicapped persons—people with one leg, or polio-crippled, even blind—who, in spite of their handicaps can truly be said to have positive good health. Yet the person whose only problem is a weight one, for example, which can be cured by just a little cutting down on food, continues to avoid taking the necessary step, and continues to be slightly unhappy about life in general.

As I read back, I have the feeling that some may mistake me for a kill-joy who wants to rob you of the pleasures of life. I certainly do not intend this. I do not advocate a return to the old Puritan days where even the simplest pleasure was frowned upon—taking a walk, for instance, if it did not contribute to the work of the community. The Puritans weren't happy people, either. They were as extreme in their withdrawals from all pleasures as the person who experiments with LSD and drugs just for the kicks.

Nor am I concerned here about social problems as such. The fire department worries about smokers because they are inclined to set buildings on fire. The social worker worries about drinking because she sees its results in broken families. The dean of the school worries about drugs because they affect the discipline. The employer is concerned about overweight because such people are often sluggish workers. The police official worries about apathetic citizens because it makes the job of law enforcement more difficult.

Husbands and wives deplore grouchy mates because it makes home life unpleasant. The church is worried about passive congregations because they fear that they are only giving lip service to their religions. And there are always some moralists with us who are unhappy about anyone who doesn't toe the line as they see it.

I speak as a doctor who has been counseling patients for more than thirty years. And my concern with these matters is only as they affect health. The unhappy fact is that the medical profession can do absolutely nothing about this great group of "minor ailers" in the country. Only they can help themselves.

Why can't they help themselves? This is the bafflement. We are supposed to have the highest level of intelligence and literacy in the history of the human race. But as far as understanding the basic rules of health—which are the same as they have always been—we are up against a stone wall. Maybe it's because the rules are so basic and obvious that we encounter resistance.

For instance, take a simple health routine like brushing your teeth. In this day and age you would think that everyone but a tiny handful of people brush their teeth at least once a day. But a recent survey by the Public Health Service states that 87 per cent is the maximum. All right, maybe that's the most we can expect. But how many, do you suppose, brush their teeth when it does most good, which is after a meal? Only 40 per cent. This shows what we're up against. Brushing teeth and other basic habits of good health are started before the school age. So if you don't want to take our simple hints for yourself, maybe at least you'll pass them on to your children.

The Basic Instincts for Good Health

The curious thing is that man is born into the world with the basic instincts for good health. If the baby has no physical ailments and his simple needs are taken care of, he is a happy and cheerful person. As he develops, nature encourages him to eat the right foods, to run and play to get stronger, to have an open mind and curiosity toward the world about him.

But man likes to tinker and he's been tinkering with his health since the beginning of time. Simply read any study of any primitive society or early civilization and you can find how man has managed, in his desire to experiment, all kinds of ridiculous, harmful, and often horrible ways of treating the human body.

Despite man's fine brain, he'd be better off observing animals to learn the basic health rules. Animals instinctively keep in good condition. They go to sleep when they're tired and get up when they've rested. They eat when hungry and they eat only enough to satisfy their appetites. And they run and romp for the sheer joy of feeling alive, and get the exercise their bodies require. Right there you have all the health rules anyone needs.

But what works for dumb animals isn't the example man seeks. Man, the superior person, has found ways to dissipate his energies, he resists his built-in health safeguards of appetite, regular sleep, and joyous, energetic play and recreation. And then he comes to the doctor to make him well again.

"I'm too smart for that plenty of sleep, fresh air, exercise routine," a patient said to me. "I don't feel well, that's all, and it's your job to do something."

Some patients are not quite as blunt but are equally frank. They say, "I don't want to live long. I just want to do what I please, and if it cuts a few years off, I don't care." Brave words, and it's your life. Yet I've visited such people in their last days, and there was not one but was willing to do anything to be given those extra years they had despised.

An Attitude Toward Life

All right, you may say, but what has all of this got to do with mental attitude? Just this. If you have your God-given cheerful outlook on life, you have no trouble in absorbing quickly and

painlessly the simple rules for good health. You accept them as
a fact of life. In current jargon, you get the message.

Now, if you don't have this attitude, how can you go about
getting it? I don't think anyone can give you a manual of in-
structions, but some hints on ways to start may be in order.

First, you have to be consciously dissatisfied with your present
way of life. To paraphrase the advertising line, if you are living
it up more and enjoying it less, you ought to figure out why this
is so.

Enjoyment is a key word. If you're not enjoying life, it is a
bad sign. You have to ask yourself some questions. What is contributing to your lack of enjoyment? Is it your job? Is it your
financial situation? Is it where you live? You'll have to sit down
with yourself and do the hard job of thinking.

Where should you think? Not at the office, not at your home.
These places have familiar associations. You need a change of
scene. Remember Bernard Baruch, who did his thinking on a park
bench? Or get on a bus or train and take a short trip to anywhere. Take a walk by the beach or in the woods.

If you are plagued with minor ailments, of course you should
have a health examination. Everyone should anyway. But the
chances are good that you have nothing seriously wrong. This is
an opportunity, however, to seek your doctor's advice. Even
though you think you know the rules of health, sometimes hearing
them again from a doctor is helpful.

Once you have determined that there is no real reason for that
persistent headache or those stomach upsets, try to forget about
it if one occurs. Resist taking that pill and go to the movies instead. Try to find some active kind of recreation that you enjoy, and
pursue it—swimming, bowling, dancing, and the like.

In Conclusion

This matter of mental attitude and health is an extremely difficult subject to communicate. People today are so accustomed to

medical advances that they expect that shots and pills will instantly cure any ailment. Yet it is true that the body functions better when a person has a positive attitude toward life. And, in mysterious ways, the person with this kind of attitude is often able to resist diseases that affect the people around him. I can tell you that this is so, but only you can learn for yourself how to benefit from this power.

Perhaps the best way for you to see that you were born with this power is to observe a small child. The ordinary, normal child enjoys himself. He likes to play, he is interested in new experiences, he is curious about everything around him. This built-in attitude encourages him to move about and grow strong. Now you don't have to stop playing when you're an adult. Thomas Hoving, for a very short time New York's Parks Commissioner, made many New Yorkers happier people. With the simple theory that parks are something people should enjoy, he provided all kinds of special events in which people could participate and have good, healthy fun.

This getting out of one's shell, enjoying things the way you did when you were a child, is one of the secrets of good health. Once you have regained that sense of wonder and curiosity about things, you will find that the rules of health will become easy to understand and to practice.

Once when I was discoursing in this vein, a friend said to me, "What about Winston Churchill? He certainly didn't follow your rules. He was overweight, he stayed up late, and he probably drank and ate and smoked more than was good for him. But he lived to a fine old age."

"He was an exception in many ways," I said, "but I think that he actually proves my point. Sir Winston Churchill had a tremendous zest for living. His enthusiasm and his enjoyment of whatever he did were boundless. And this is undoubtedly the reason that he was able to surmount a regimen of life that would have felled a more passive person much earlier."

My friend pursued the point. "Do you mean, then," he asked,

"that if I cultivate this cheerful, positive attitude I'll live to be as old as Churchill?"

My answer to him—and to you—is this: "Not necessarily, but you'll have more fun."

20. How to Retire
and Be Happy

Retirement should be a happy reward for many years of work. Will this be true for you?

Only recently a businessman came to see me upon the eve of his retirement. For the past six months, he said, he had been restless and irritable and progressively alarmed about the rapidly approaching day when he would leave his desk for the final time. That event, he predicted, would be to him like the last walk of a condemned prisoner to the electric chair. He had three worries— the three elements that affect all of us in facing retirement:

Money: Would he be able to adjust to a reduced income? He had only recently figured out his pension and social security and realized that the drop from his salary would be considerable.

Time: How would he fill all of the empty hours? All he had lived for was the job. He had no outside interests.

Health: Would he suddenly collapse physically and spend his last years in a wheel chair?

I would like to say that I was able to offer some help which got him back on the track. Actually, all I could do was give him a health examination and assure him that he was not in danger of a collapse. But nothing could be done about his financial situation or his attitude toward leisure time.

This man had waited too long. He had not prepared himself for what he had long known was an inevitable event. He may become one of the less happy oldsters because of the lack of foresight.

But retirement need not be this way. I think by contrast of another friend whose retirement dinner I attended last year. "John," I said, "what is the first thing you are going to do the day you leave your office for good?" John brightened. "I figured that out years ago," he said. "I'm going to start walking in any direction I like. Because for the first time in my life I'll be a free man— there are so many things I want to do."

This is the correct attitude, of course, and John will have few retirement problems because he began his preparation years ago. So, if you are on the verge of retirement and dread it, don't be too disturbed. If you are blessed with reasonably good health and adequate retirement income, you will cultivate interests that will be consistent with your income. But if you are as little as five years or as many as thirty years away from retirement, there are some steps you can take now that will help give you greater assurance of the happy retirement you deserve. Life itself is preparation. From birth on we prepare for the careers we should follow, and retirement is simply another career.

Unfortunately, many people seem unable to bring themselves to facing up to this. The three basic worries that needled my businessman friend are often stumbling blocks.

Health, of course, is my interest, but the two other factors, money and what you will do with your time, have a bearing on health and are critical to a successful retirement. The three factors are, in fact, interdependent. Without sufficient money, for instance, retirement may become a tragedy. Without good health, retirement can be miserable. But even with sufficient money and a good physical condition, you will not be happy unless you have something meaningful to do with your time.

So let's review these factors in more detail.

Money for Retirement

Will you have enough money for retirement? The financing of retirement is an American invention. Private pension plans plus social security give increasing millions of families assurance that they will be able to live comfortably, if not in style. Already, for many people, retirement income will be considerably more than bare subsistence. But, with inflation and temptation to do more interesting things such as travel, it is wise to put aside as much extra as you can. Be realistic about the value of money. $100,000 seems like a lot of money to most of us. Yet if you have to live on the income from $100,000 you will be able to afford only the bare necessities. Being financially secure in retirement years gives you the necessary peace of mind that will make your retirement more enjoyable—and more healthful. A good mental attitude, and freedom from worry, is bound to benefit your health.

I am no financial expert, but facing up to your money situation is the first step in planning a successful retirement. Reviewing your insurance is an obvious step also in planning retirement. If you are purchasing an annuity, make sure the rate of return is as good as investing in blue chip stocks. Look into health insurance, which you may need to augment Medicare benefits. Don't forget that despite Medicare hospital charges continue to rise and will do so for some time to come. We are not suggesting that you worry about the possibility of needing hospitalization. It is simply prudent to protect yourself in case the need arises.

Even though you think you know you'll have a good-sized pension, it's wise to start your own investment program. There are few people who can't use additional money once retirement starts.

What Will You Do?

Assuming that you are reasonably sure of a good financial situation when you retire, the big question then becomes, what will you do with this bonus time? Most people today can count on ten to fourteen years after a retirement at sixty-five. In human terms this is a long time, particularly when you realize that the hours you now devote to working and preparing for work each day will become yours.

If you are a person with many outside interests, you should have little to worry about in using this extra time. But if you devote yourself only to your job and simply watch TV at night for recreation, you are heading for trouble. You can't watch TV all day long. So now is the time to expand your interests, to plan some projects of your own—and try to make them active projects. (The reason for this will be discussed later.)

It is to meet this very well-recognized need that John W. Gardner, Secretary of Health, Education and Welfare, is proposing "mid-career clinics," places where men and women could go "to re-examine the goals of their working life and consider changes of direction."

"All too often the man reaching age 65 has spent much of his work career in a routine of blind alley job, has been denied the opportunity to think actively and constructively about the use of his abilities and has learned no new skills or interests for years," Mr. Gardner said recently. "Then we plunge him into one of life's toughest adjustments and expect him to make it easily."

I was glad to note that the Secretary also added that people should be given a choice on what they want to do. This is why he urges that these retirement clinics be started at least ten or fifteen years before retirement to give a person a chance to figure out what is best for him.

Whatever you decide to do, and however you do it, keep in

mind the problems of your wife. While you and your spouse may have been having daydreams together about that great day when the two of you would have time to become reacquainted, the reality may be shocking. After a few weeks, you may find that there is really not much to discuss with your wife. And, more humiliating, you may find that your devoted wife is a bit uneasy about having you around the house disrupting a routine she has been following for forty years or so. So, in your retirement planning, allow some time for both of you to have some privacy. And the more outside interests your wife develops that she can continue in retirement, the better both of you will be.

What you should both be seeking in retirement is not an open end vacation, but another kind of a career. A vacation means a change—that's why it's good for you and is enjoyable. So if you think of retirement as a career in itself, and continue to take vacations from this new career, you will be better off.

Your Health

But even if you have all of the money you need and all of the interests to keep you busy, your health is still the most important factor. In fact, it is fear of failing health that worries many people about retirement. Some patients have told me that retirement day to them means an immediate decline in health. The folklore is full of stories about men dropping dead six months after retirement, or moving into nursing homes where they deteriorate rapidly.

This is a lot of nonsense. Physical deterioration starts with adulthood. The person who has a physical collapse shortly after retirement would have had it if he had continued working. Whatever his ailment, if started years before. So, in your planning for retirement, give some attention to your present state of health.

It is true that having sufficient money and something to occupy you will be beneficial to your health. But your actual condition now, assuming you are five to twenty years away from retirement, will be a good clue as to how healthy you will be in your later years.

A thorough physical examination now is an obvious requisite. But, assuming that nothing serious is found, you should have a long talk with your doctor about habits of living which may be taking a long-range toll.

The various points we have tried to make in past chapters—on the heart, on overweight, on smoking, on exercise, use of leisure time—are all directed to extending your life and giving you a happy retirement.

It is well and good that older people can be provided with adequate medical care without breaking their budgets. However, many of the tragic cases of physical collapse in later years need not have happened. It is the prevention of disease and disability which we always advocate, and this approach to health in early years will be the payoff in retirement.

The fifty-year-old who has trouble walking up stairs or walking around the block may not be in shape at retirement to even take a boat trip. The overweight person who reaches retirement is going to find a number of "minor" ailments creeping up that may make retirement an unpleasant experience. All of which reminds me of a patient who told me she was looking forward to old age because she would begin at last to lose weight. Her reason for this belief was based on the fact that one rarely sees a very old person who is overweight. It was my unhappy duty to explain that, while her observation was correct, the reason is that overweight people don't live to be very old.

Among other preventive steps that should be taken into middle age is care of the teeth, eyes, and hearing. Many old people today, living on small incomes, have difficulty in affording dental care, glasses, and hearing aids. And they are not provided for by Medicare. Again, the answer is in taking care of these precious assets in middle age as difficulties arise.

Often, when discussing this situation, I am asked about the special health problems of the aged. The health problems of the geriattric age are no different from those of younger people. Prevention of health problems is still the best solution. Whether twenty-one, forty-one, or eighty-one we are all subject to the same stresses and the same dangers. No one dies of old age. We all die from a specific cause—a disease, an accident, or the degeneration of some important organs of the body.

Recently a friend of mine was discussing his parents. His mother had died in her late sixties of multiple ailments, while his father, in his eighties, was still going strong. My friend pointed out that the couple had both been vigorous in their youth. "Why the difference?" he asked. First, heredity is very important.

I asked him to answer a few questions as follows:

"Was your mother overweight?"

"Yes, most of her adult life."

"Did your mother have a strong interest in life?"

"No."

"Was this true of your father?"

"No. He took long walks every day—still does—kept down his weight, had many interests. In fact, when he retired, he taught himself Latin."

"No further questions," I said. "You've found the answer."

Some Pitfalls to Avoid

To some people, retirement means moving to Florida or California. While many of them make a successful adjustment to this uprooting process, a number of them regret it. The wise approach, I believe, is not to be too hasty in selling your house and taking the plunge. Instead, go for about three months. Rent a house rather than staying at a hotel. And go in the off season. Then, if you wish you were back home in the familiar community where you lived, you can return without difficulty. Women, I have noted, often find it hard to adjust to a new community. So make sure your wife has her say before you move.

An acquaintance of mine is approaching this problem wisely, I think. He and his wife got the notion that it would be enjoyable to live in London for the first year of their retirement, not in a hotel, but in an apartment. The planning of this venture has given them something in common and they are looking at retirement day as an opportunity to do something they both want. But a year is a long time, so they are first going on an eight-week charter flight to explore the situation. And if they find that life in London doesn't seem as appealing close up, they have not committed themselves.

I am also asked about retirement communities. A number of people seem to like them because of the many services provided, the recreational and medical facilities, the association with persons with common interests. But others have told me that they find such communities, with no young people about, to be depressing. Only you can decide which it would be for you. So investigate carefully before you act.

Should Retirement Be Mandatory?

A mandatory retirement, generally at sixty-five, is certainly to be recommended. In fact, I believe that there should be a mandatory retirement for congressmen, senators, and other government officials with important responsibilities. This is the only orderly way in which our society can operate, and individuals are happier, too, if they know the rules of the game. People should be conditioned early in life that retirement will come, that they are not supposed to hang on indefinitely.

This doesn't mean that a person can't start a second career if he so chooses—and it's something he wants to do—not a time filler. I recall a dramatic case a few years ago. It concerned a ninety-year-old man retiring after twenty-five years with an accounting firm. I found that at sixty-five he had retired from a corporation where he held a routine job. But, going to night school, he had learned accounting. And, on retirement day he started a completely new career. I don't necessarily advocate this. The important point in this case is that this man wanted to do what he did—it made him happy—and that's what counts.

What kinds of people seem to adjust best to retirement? The answer is, those who have multiple interests, who enjoy life and strive to do as many different things as possible. Put another way, the person who is happy now is likely to be happy in retirement.

What about the top executive who manages a big enterprise? Won't he lose that sense of power when he suddenly retires? In theory, yes, but many such executives I have met find plenty of other ways to release their energies. I think, for instance, of Clarence Randall, who retired as chairman of the board of Inland Steel in 1952. Since then he has held important government positions and just recently I saw a copy of a book he has written.

In fact, one reason for a mandatory retirement is that the country benefits from the additional enterprises engaged in by retired executives. A Clarence Randall, if he had continued in his job, would never have had the time to lend his talents to the government or share his wisdom through books. And the men behind him would have been frustrated in reaching the top.

As I observe all of the complicated problems faced by our society—all of the important jobs yet unfinished—I believe we should seek new ways to enlist the talents of our retired citizens. Many executives today are trying to carry too big a load. In addition to their exacting jobs, they participate in all kinds of public service activities that take them away from the office and from their homes. The more these public service activities can be handled by retired persons, the more we'll all benefit—and it will give the retirees a sense of purpose. I also believe that those who want to work after retirement and are competent should not be discriminated against because of age. Many studies have shown that older workers are often more reliable and productive than the very young.

The Crucial Decades—Forty-five to Sixty-five

The most crucial period toward a happy retirement is between the ages of forty-five to sixty-five.

This is when a man is at the height of his powers and can really comprehend modern America, the interesting things to do, and the multiple problems to be solved. As he begins to realize that there are many things in this world other than his own job, he will unconsciously be preparing himself for new explorations when retirement day comes.

Unfortunately, this is the period when men are vulnerable to the degenerative diseases that plague modern America.

Coronary heart disease, the Number One killer, hits primarily men after age forty-five. The odds are that you will live at least fourteen more years after you reach sixty-five. But your first objective has to be to reach sixty-five. This is why we urge so vigorously the development of sound health practices for the middle-aged. What you do in the crucial decades will largely determine whether you reach retirement age—and, if you do, how healthy a retirement you will enjoy.

These are the years when you should take a complete inventory of your financial assets, your interest in life, and your physical condition. When you get your annual health checkup, have a talk with your doctor about your health routine. Have him guide you in firmly establishing a regimen of weight control and sufficient exercise. At the same time re-examine smoking (a major factor in heart disease) and alcohol consumption, which contributes, at the very least, to overweight problems.

Get a life pattern established in these crucial years to get you to retirement day, and then retirement will not be the problem you may now think it is.

Retirement Preparation—an Example

A remarkable organization called the Telephone Pioneers illustrates the points I have been making about retirement preparation. Formed within the A T & T system in 1911, it has more than two hundred thousand members all over the country. It is not an organization of retired persons, as you might think. Rather, after a person completes twenty-one years of employment, he becomes a member of the Pioneers. Since the Bell System usually hires only young people, this means that most persons are in their forties when they join. They continue as members for life. So when they attend the many meetings and social events that are offered, the age range can be from forty to eighty.

Thus the forty-year-old becomes subtly aware that one day he will retire and that it won't be traumatic. And the eighty-year-old finds himself still a member of the company, mixing with younger people, keeping in touch with what is going on.

Without being rigid, the Pioneer program provides a vehicle for retirement preparation. There are investment clinics where the younger person can learn about ways to handle money. There is a variety of other programs such as travel to nearby historical spots, theater parties, even Mediterranean cruises, all of which develop a variety of interests. And through an industrial health program and annual examinations, the Pioneers learn the importance of health.

This kind of program gives the preparation needed, yet a person is not viewing retirement as something alarming. Rather it becomes a pleasant prospect.

But few companies can provide such an elaborate setup. What can you do if you are not working for a large organization and hence have no access to such facilities?

The libraries and bookstores are full of material on investment planning. Many brokerage houses offer free courses, and there are such courses available in schools and colleges.

If you lead a normal social life and if you take advantage of the cultural and sports opportunities wherever you live, you will develop the interests that you will want to pursue when retired. Doubtless you have said to yourself occasionally that if you "only had the time," you would learn a foreign language, a musical instrument, etc. Retirement is going to give you that time you've been asking for. Just be ready.

And if your company does not provide health examinations and counsel, you can obtain these from a doctor or health clinic.

Does Retirement Work?

You may well say at this point, "All right, what you say seems to make sense. But does anyone really know whether retired people who have followed such a program of preparation are really happy with their lot."

As far as I can tell, not much has been done to test the results of retirement preparation. We made a study of our own a few years ago, through the Life Extension Foundation, which I believe is still pertinent. It was national in scope and covered 1500 retired persons in manufacturing, banking, advertising, retailing, wholesaling, and the service fields. Prior to retirement, their jobs had ranged from positions in top management to office, clerical and factory duties. Over half had been retired one to five years; over a third, five or more years; and the small balance less than one year. They represented a wide range of economic levels.

On the whole, the results were encouraging. Only 11 per cent said that their routine was boring, only 17 per cent said that they did not feel as well as before, and 27 per cent said they felt better. However, the matter of money seemed to be an important factor; 460 out of the 1500 replied that they wished they were back at their old jobs. But 84 per cent of those responding in this way were in the lowest income bracket—well under $5000 a year. I think we can assume that it was the income they missed, not the job itself. Perhaps the executive level better prepared themselves for retirement—more hobbies etc.—while the lower income group had few interests and really missed the job, as menial as it was.

From this study we verified that financial preparation and the early establishment of good health habits (the 1500 were selected from those who had regular health examinations during their working years) are important keys to a happy retirement. With good health and sufficient income, most people learn to adjust to the extra time on their hands.

We also learned through this survey experience that the first year of retirement is the critical one. It is significant, I think, that many top executives found the first year particularly difficult, while employees at a lower level adjusted better. However, after the second year, almost the reverse was true. Here again I believe it is because the lower level group begins to experience financial difficulties, while the executive group, financially secure, has begun to use its talents in various outside activities.

Conclusions

•The three main elements in a happy retirement are sufficient income, keeping busy with things you like to do, and good health.
•You can't start too early in planning for retirement, but you don't have to go about it in a formal way.
•If you plan your financial affairs wisely, you will have sufficient income.
•If you develop outside interests besides your office and family life, you will have no problem with too much time on your hands.
•If you develop good health habits at least by middle age, the chances are that you will enjoy another fourteen years after retirement. Keep in mind the "crucial years"—forty-five to sixty-five,

the period when you set the pattern—financial, outside interest, and health—that will carry you through to retirement day.

•If you've done these things, retirement won't sneak up on you by surprise. It will be a natural, pleasant event, as natural as graduating from school and pleasant for the prospect of many good years to come.

Appendix

The Nutritive Value of 500 Common Foods

Item No.	Food and approximate measure		Food Energy	Pro-tein	Fat (total lipid)	Car-bohy-drate
	MILK, CREAM, CHEESE; RELATED PRODUCTS		*Calo-ries*	*Gm.*	*Gm.*	*Gm.*
	Milk, cow's:					
1	Fluid, whole (3.5% fat)	1 cup	160	9	9	12
2	Fluid, nonfat (skim)	1 cup	90	9	Trace	13
3	Buttermilk, cultured, from skim milk	1 cup	90	9	Trace	13
4	Evaporated, unsweetened, undiluted	1 cup	345	18	20	24
5	Condensed, sweetened, undiluted	1 cup	980	25	27	166
6	Dry, whole	1 cup	515	27	28	39

This table of nutritive values for common household measures of foods was prepared by the home economists of the United States Department of Agriculture. This is the second edition of the table, revised in 1964.

Item No.	Food and approximate measure		Food Energy	Protein	Fat (total lipid)	Carbohydrate
	MILK, CREAM, CHEESE; RELATED PRODUCTS—Cont'd		*Calories*	*Gm.*	*Gm.*	*Gm.*
	Milk, cow's—continued					
7	Dry, nonfat, instant	1 cup	250	25	Trace	36
	Milk, goat's:					
8	Fluid, whole	1 cup	165	8	10	11
	Cream:					
9	Half-and-half	1 cup	325	8	28	11
10	(cream and milk)	1 tablespoon	20	Trace	2	1
11	Light (coffee or	1 cup	505	7	49	10
12	table)	1 tablespoon	30	Trace	3	1
	Whipping, unwhipped (volume about double when whipped):					
13	Light	1 cup	715	6	75	9
14		1 tablespoon	45	Trace	5	1
15	Heavy	1 cup	840	5	89	7
16		1 tablespoon	55	Trace	6	Trace
	Cheese:					
17	Blue or Roquefort	1 ounce	105	6	9	1
	Cheddar or American:					
18	Ungrated	1 inch cube	70	4	5	Trace
19	Grated	1 cup	445	28	36	2
20		1 tablespoon	30	2	2	Trace
21	Cheddar, process	1 ounce	105	7	9	1
22	Cheese foods, Cheddar	1 ounce	90	6	7	2
	Cottage cheese, from skim milk:					
23	Creamed	1 cup	240	31	9	7
24		1 ounce	30	4	1	1
25	Uncreamed	1 cup	195	38	1	6
26		1 ounce	25	5	Trace	1
27	Cream cheese	1 ounce	105	2	11	1
28		1 tablespoon	55	1	6	Trace
29	Swiss (domestic)	1 ounce	105	8	8	1
	Milk beverages:					
30	Cocoa	1 cup	235	9	11	26

Item No.	Food and approximate measure		Food Energy	Pro-tein	Fat (total lipid)	Car-bohy-drate
	MILK, CREAM, CHEESE; RELATED PRODUCTS—Cont'd		*Calo-ries*	*Gm.*	*Gm.*	*Gm.*
	Milk beverages—continued					
31	Chocolate-flavored milk drink (made with skim milk)	1 cup	190	8	6	27
32	Malted milk	1 cup	280	13	12	32
	Milk desserts:					
33	Cornstarch pud-ding, plain (blanc mange)	1 cup	275	9	10	39
34	Custard, baked	1 cup	285	13	14	28
	Ice cream, plain, factory packed:					
35	Slice or cut brick, $\frac{1}{8}$ of quart brick	1 slice or cut brick	145	3	9	15
36	Container	$3\frac{1}{2}$ fluid ounces	130	2	8	13
37	Container	8 fluid ounces	295	6	18	29
38	Ice milk	1 cup	285	9	10	42
39	Yoghurt, from partially skimmed milk	1 cup	120	8	4	13
	EGGS					
	Eggs, large, 24 ounces per dozen: Raw:					
40	Whole, without shell	1 egg	80	6	6	Trace
41	White of egg	1 white	15	4	Trace	Trace
42	Yolk of egg	1 yolk	60	3	5	Trace
	Cooked:					
43	Boiled, shell removed	2 eggs	160	13	12	1
44	Scrambled, with milk and fat	1 egg	110	7	8	1

Item No.	Food and approximate measure		Food Energy	Protein	Fat (total lipid)	Carbohydrate
	MEAT, POULTRY, FISH, SHELLFISH; RELATED PRODUCTS		Calories	Gm.	Gm.	Gm.
45	Bacon, broiled or fried, crisp	2 slices	100	5	8	1
	Beef, trimmed to retail basis, cooked:					
	Cuts braised, simmered, or pot-roasted:					
46	Lean and fat	3 ounces	245	23	16	0
47	Lean only	2.5 ounces	140	22	5	0
	Hamburger (ground beef), broiled:					
48	Lean	3 ounces	185	23	10	0
49	Regular	3 ounces	245	21	17	0
	Roast, oven-cooked, no liquid added:					
	Relatively fat, such as rib:					
50	Lean and fat	3 ounces	375	17	34	0
51	Lean only	1.8 ounces	125	14	7	0
	Relatively lean, such as heel of round:					
52	Lean and fat	3 ounces	165	25	7	0
53	Lean only	2.7 ounces	125	24	3	0
	Steak, broiled:					
	Relatively fat, such as sirloin:					
54	Lean and fat	3 ounces	330	20	27	0
55	Lean only	2.0 ounces	115	18	4	0
	Relatively lean, such as round:					
56	Lean and fat	3 ounces	220	24	13	0
57	Lean only	2.4 ounces	130	21	4	0
	Beef, canned:					
58	Corned beef	3 ounces	185	22	10	0
59	Corned beef hash	3 ounces	155	7	10	9
60	Beef, dried or chipped	2 ounces	115	19	4	0
61	Beef-vegetable stew	1 cup	210	15	10	15

Item No.	Food and approximate measure		Food Energy	Protein	Fat (total lipid)	Carbohydrate
	MEAT, POULTRY, FISH, SHELLFISH; RELATED PRODUCTS—Cont'd		*Calories*	*Gm.*	*Gm.*	*Gm.*
62	Beef potpie, baked: 1 pie Individual pie, 4¼-inch diameter, weight before baking about 8 ounces		560	23	33	43
	Chicken, cooked:					
63	Flesh only, broiled 3 ounces		115	20	3	0
	Breast, fried, ½ breast:					
64	With bone	3.3 ounces	155	25	5	1
65	Flesh and skin	2.7 ounces	155	25	5	1
	Drumstick, fried:					
66	With bone	2.1 ounces	90	12	4	Trace
67	Flesh and skin	1.3 ounces	90	12	4	Trace
68	Chicken, canned, boneless	3 ounces	170	18	10	0
	Chicken potpie. *See* Poultry potpie					
	Chile con carne; canned:					
69	With beans	1 cup	335	19	15	30
70	Without beans	1 cup	510	26	38	15
71	Heart, beef, lean, braised	3 ounces	160	27	5	1
	Lamb, trimmed to retail basis, cooked:					
72	Chop, thick, with bone, broiled.	1 chop 4.8 ounces	400	25	33	0
73	Lean and fat	4.0 ounces	400	25	33	0
74	Lean only	2.6 ounces	140	21	6	0
	Leg, roasted:					
75	Lean and fat	3 ounces	235	22	16	0
76	Lean only	2.5 ounces	130	20	5	0
	Shoulder, roasted:					
77	Lean and fat	3 ounces	285	18	23	0
78	Lean only	2.3 ounces	130	17	6	0
79	Liver, beef, fried	2 ounces	130	15	6	3

Item No.	Food and approximate measure		Food Energy	Protein	Fat (total lipid)	Carbohydrate
	MEAT, POULTRY, FISH, SHELLFISH; RELATED PRODUCTS—Cont'd		*Calories*	*Gm.*	*Gm.*	*Gm.*
	Pork, cured, cooked:					
80	Ham, light cure, lean and fat, roasted	3 ounces	245	18	19	0
	Luncheon meat:					
81	Boiled ham, sliced	2 ounces	135	11	10	0
82	Canned, spiced or unspiced	2 ounces	165	8	14	1
	Pork, fresh, trimmed to retail basis, cooked:					
83	Chop, thick, with bone	1 chop, 3.5 ounces	260	16	21	0
84	Lean and fat	2.3 ounces	260	16	21	0
85	Lean only	1.7 ounces	130	15	7	0
	Roast, oven-cooked, no liquid added:					
86	Lean and fat	3 ounces	310	21	24	0
87	Lean only	2.4 ounces	175	20	10	0
	Cuts, simmered:					
88	Lean and fat	3 ounces	320	20	26	0
89	Lean only	2.2 ounces	135	18	6	0
90	Poultry potpie (based on chicken potpie). Individual pie, $4\frac{1}{4}$-inch diameter, weight before baking about 8 ounces	1 pie	535	23	31	42
	Sausage:					
91	Bologna, slice, 4.1 by 0.1 inch	8 slices	690	27	62	2
92	Frankfurter, cooked	1 frankfurter	155	6	14	1
93	Pork, links or patty, cooked	4 ounces	540	21	50	Trace
94	Tongue, beef, braised	3 ounces	210	18	14	Trace

Item No.	Food and approximate measure		Food Energy	Protein	Fat (total lipid)	Carbohydrate
	MEAT, POULTRY, FISH, SHELLFISH; RELATED PRODUCTS—Cont'd		Calories	Gm.	Gm.	Gm.
	Turkey potpie. *See* Poultry potpie					
	Veal, cooked:					
95	Cutlet, without bone, broiled	3 ounces	185	23	9	–
96	Roast, medium fat, medium done; lean and fat	3 ounces	230	23	14	0
	Fish and shellfish:					
97	Bluefish, baked or broiled	3 ounces	135	22	4	0
	Clams:					
98	Raw, meat only	3 ounces	65	11	1	2
99	Canned, solids and liquid	3 ounces	45	7	1	2
100	Crabmeat, canned	3 ounces	85	15	2	1
101	Fish sticks, breaded, cooked, frozen; stick, 3.8 by 1.0 by 0.5 inch	10 sticks or 8-ounce package	400	38	20	15
102	Haddock, fried	3 ounces	140	17	5	5
	Mackerel:					
103	Broiled, Atlantic	3 ounces	200	19	13	0
104	Canned, Pacific, solids and liquid	3 ounces	155	18	9	0
105	Ocean perch, breaded (egg and breadcrumbs), fried	3 ounces	195	16	11	6
106	Oysters, meat only: Raw, 13–19 medium selects	1 cup	160	20	4	8
107	Oyster stew, 1 part oysters to 3 parts milk by volume, 3–4 oysters	1 cup	200	11	12	11
108	Salmon, pink, canned	3 ounces	120	17	5	0

Item No.	Food and approximate measure	Food Energy	Protein	Fat (total lipid)	Carbohydrate
	MEAT, POULTRY, FISH, SHELLFISH; RELATED PRODUCTS—Cont'd	Calories	Gm.	Gm.	Gm.
	Fish and shellfish—continued				
109	Sardines, Atlantic, 3 ounces canned in oil, drained solids	175	20	9	0
110	Shad, baked 3 ounces	170	20	10	0
111	Shrimp, canned, 3 ounces meat only	100	21	1	1
112	Swordfish, 3 ounces broiled with butter or margarine	150	24	5	0
113	Tuna, canned in 3 ounces oil, drained solids	170	24	7	0
	MATURE DRY BEANS AND PEAS, NUTS, PEANUTS; RELATED PRODUCTS				
114	Almonds, shelled 1 cup	850	26	77	28
	Beans, dry:				
	Common varieties, such as Great Northern, navy, and others, canned:				
115	Red 1 cup	230	15	1	42
	White, with tomato sauce:				
116	With pork 1 cup	320	16	7	50
117	Without pork 1 cup	310	16	1	60
118	Lima, cooked 1 cup	260	16	1	48
119	Brazil nuts 1 cup	915	20	94	15
120	Cashew nuts, roasted 1 cup	760	23	62	40
	Coconut:				
121	Fresh, shredded 1 cup	335	3	34	9
122	Dried, shredded, sweetened 1 cup	340	2	24	33

Item No.	Food and approximate measure		Food Energy	Protein	Fat (total lipid)	Carbohydrate
	MATURE DRY BEANS AND PEAS, NUTS, PEANUTS; RELATED PRODUCTS—Cont'd					
			Calories	*Gm.*	*Gm.*	*Gm.*
123	Cowpeas or black-eye peas, dry, cooked	1 cup	190	13	1	34
	Peanuts, roasted, salted:					
124	Halves	1 cup	840	37	72	27
125	Chopped	1 tablespoon	55	2	4	2
126	Peanut butter	1 tablespoon	95	4	8	3
127	Peas, split, dry, cooked	1 cup	290	20	1	52
	Pecans:					
128	Halves	1 cup	740	10	77	16
129	Chopped	1 tablespoon	50	1	5	1
	Walnuts, shelled:					
130	Black or native, chopped	1 cup	790	26	75	19
	English or Persian:					
131	Halves	1 cup	650	15	64	16
132	Chopped	1 tablespoon	50	1	5	1
	VEGETABLES AND VEGETABLE PRODUCTS					
	Asparagus:					
133	Cooked, cut spears	1 cup	35	4	Trace	6
	Canned spears, medium:					
134	Green	6 spears	20	2	Trace	3
135	Bleached	6 spears	20	2	Trace	4
	Beans:					
136	Lima, immature, cooked	1 cup	180	12	1	32
	Snap, green:					
	Cooked:					
137	Small amount of water, short time	1 cup	30	2	Trace	7

Item No.	Food and approximate measure		Food Energy	Protein	Fat (total lipid)	Carbohydrate
	VEGETABLES AND VEGETABLE PRODUCTS—Cont'd		*Calories*	*Gm.*	*Gm.*	*Gm.*
	Beans—continued					
	Snap, green:					
	Cooked:					
138	Large amount of water, long time	1 cup	30	2	Trace	7
	Canned:					
139	Solids and liquid	1 cup	45	2	Trace	10
140	Strained or chopped (baby food)	1 ounce	5	Trace	Trace	1
	Bean sprouts. *See* Sprouts					
141	Beets, cooked, diced	1 cup	50	2	Trace	12
142	Broccoli spears, cooked	1 cup	40	5	Trace	7
143	Brussels sprouts, cooked	1 cup	45	5	1	8
	Cabbage:					
	Raw:					
144	Finely shredded	1 cup	25	1	Trace	5
145	Coleslaw	1 cup	120	1	9	9
	Cooked:					
146	Small amount of water, short time	1 cup	35	2	Trace	7
147	Large amount of water, long time	1 cup	30	2	Trace	7
	Cabbage, celery or Chinese:					
148	Raw, leaves and stalk, 1-inch pieces	1 cup	15	1	Trace	3
149	Cabbage, spoon (or pakchoy), cooked	1 cup	20	2	Trace	4
	Carrots:					
	Raw:					
150	Whole, $5\frac{1}{2}$ by 1 inch, (25 thin strips)	1 carrot	20	1	Trace	5

Item No.	Food and approximate measure		Food Energy	Pro- tein	Fat (total lipid)	Car- bohy- drate
	VEGETABLES AND VEGETABLE PRODUCTS—Cont'd		Calo- ries	Gm.	Gm.	Gm.
	Carrots—continued Raw:					
151	Grated	1 cup	45	1	Trace	11
152	Cooked, diced	1 cup	45	1	Trace	10
153	Canned, strained or chopped (baby food)	1 ounce	10	Trace	Trace	2
154	Cauliflower, cooked, flowerbuds	1 cup	25	3	Trace	5
	Celery, raw:					
155	Stalk, large outer, 8 by about $1\frac{1}{2}$ inches, at root end	1 stalk	5	Trace	Trace	2
156	Pieces, diced	1 cup	15	1	Trace	4
157	Collards, cooked	1 cup	55	5	1	9
	Corn, sweet:					
158	Cooked, ear 5 by $1\frac{3}{4}$ inches	1 ear	70	3	1	16
159	Canned, solids and liquid	1 cup	170	5	2	40
160	Cowpeas, cooked, immature seeds	1 cup	175	13	1	29
	Cucumbers, 10-ounce; $7\frac{1}{2}$ by about 2 inches:					
161	Raw, pared	1 cucumber	30	1	Trace	7
162	Raw, pared, center slice $\frac{1}{8}$-inch thick	6 slices	5	Trace	Trace	2
163	Dandelion greens, cooked	1 cup	60	4	1	12
164	Endive, curly (in- cluding escarole)	2 ounces	10	1	Trace	2
165	Kale, leaves includ- ing stems, cooked	1 cup	30	4	1	4

Item No.	Food and approximate measure		Food Energy	Protein	Fat (total lipid)	Carbohydrate
	VEGETABLES AND VEGETABLE PRODUCTS—Cont'd		*Calories*	*Gm.*	*Gm.*	*Gm.*
	Lettuce, raw:					
166	Butterhead, as Boston types; head, 4-inch diameter	1 head	30	3	Trace	6
167	Crisphead, as iceberg; head, $4\frac{3}{4}$-inch diameter	1 head	60	4	Trace	13
168	Looseleaf, or bunching varieties, leaves	2 large	10	1	Trace	2
169	Mushrooms, canned, solids and liquid	1 cup	40	5	Trace	6
170	Mustard greens, cooked	1 cup	35	3	1	6
171	Okra, cooked, pod 3 by $\frac{5}{8}$ inch	8 pods	25	2	Trace	5
	Onions:					
	Mature:					
172	Raw, onion $2\frac{1}{2}$-inch diameter	1 onion	40	2	Trace	10
173	Cooked	1 cup	60	3	Trace	14
174	Young, green, small, without tops	6 onions	20	1	Trace	5
175	Parsley, raw, chopped	1 tablespoon	1	Trace	Trace	Trace
176	Parsnips, cooked	1 cup	100	2	1	23
	Peas, green:					
177	Cooked	1 cup	115	9	1	19
178	Canned, solids and liquid	1 cup	165	9	1	31
179	Canned, strained (baby food)	1 ounce	15	1	Trace	3
180	Peppers, hot, red, without seeds, dried (ground chili powder, added seasonings)	1 tablespoon	50	2	2	8

Item No.	Food and approximate measure		Food Energy	Pro-tein	Fat (total lipid)	Car-bohy-drate
	VEGETABLES AND VEGETABLE PRODUCTS—Cont'd		Calo-ries	Gm.	Gm.	Gm.
	Peppers, sweet:					
	Raw, medium, about 6 per pound:					
181	Green pod with-out stem and seeds	1 pod	15	1	Trace	3
182	Red pod without stem and seeds	1 pod	20	1	Trace	4
183	Canned, pimien-tos, medium	1 pod	10	Trace	Trace	2
	Potatoes, medium (about 3 per pound raw):					
184	Baked, peeled after baking	1 potato	90	3	Trace	21
	Boiled:					
185	Peeled after boiling	1 potato	105	3	Trace	23
186	Peeled before boiling	1 potato	80	2	Trace	18
	French-fried, piece 2 by $\frac{1}{2}$ by $\frac{1}{2}$ inch:					
187	Cooked in deep fat	10 pieces	155	2	7	20
188	Frozen, heated	10 pieces	125	2	5	19
	Mashed:					
189	Milk added	1 cup	125	4	1	25
190	Milk and butter added	1 cup	185	4	8	24
191	Potato chips, medium, 2-inch diameter	10 chips	115	1	8	10
192	Pumpkin, canned	1 cup	75	2	1	18
193	Radishes, raw, small, without tops	4 radishes	5	Trace	Trace	1
194	Sauerkraut, canned, solids and liquid	1 cup	45	2	Trace	9
	Spinach:					
195	Cooked	1 cup	40	5	1	6

Item No.	Food and approximate measure		Food Energy	Protein	Fat (total lipid)	Carbohydrate
	VEGETABLES AND VEGETABLE PRODUCTS—Cont'd		*Calories*	*Gm.*	*Gm.*	*Gm.*
	Spinach—continued					
196	Canned, drained solids	1 cup	45	5	1	6
197	Canned, strained or chopped (baby food)	1 ounce	10	1	Trace	2
	Sprouts, raw:					
198	Mung bean	1 cup	30	3	Trace	6
199	Soybean	1 cup	40	6	2	4
	Squash:					
	Cooked:					
200	Summer, diced	1 cup	30	2	Trace	7
201	Winter, baked, mashed	1 cup	130	4	1	32
202	Canned, winter, strained and chopped (baby food)	1 ounce	10	Trace	Trace	2
	Sweet potatoes:					
	Cooked, medium, 5 by 2 inches, weight raw about 6 ounces:					
203	Baked, peeled after baking	1 sweet potato	155	2	1	36
204	Boiled, peeled after boiling	1 sweet potato	170	2	1	39
205	Candied, 3½ by 2¼ inches	1 sweet potato	295	2	6	60
206	Canned, vacuum or solid pack	1 cup	235	4	Trace	54
	Tomatoes:					
207	Raw, medium, 2 by 2½ inches, about 3 per pound	1 tomato	35	2	Trace	7
208	Canned	1 cup	50	2	Trace	10
209	Tomato juice, canned	1 cup	45	2	Trace	10
210	Tomato catsup	1 tablespoon	15	Trace	Trace	4

Item No.	Food and approximate measure		Food Energy	Pro-tein	Fat (total lipid)	Car-bohy-drate
	VEGETABLES AND VEGETABLE PRODUCTS—Cont'd		*Calo-ries*	*Gm.*	*Gm.*	*Gm.*
211	Turnips, cooked, diced	1 cup	35	1	Trace	8
	Turnip greens: Cooked:					
212	In small amount of water, short time	1 cup	30	3	Trace	5
213	In large amount of water, long time	1 cup	25	3	Trace	5
214	Canned, solids and liquid	1 cup	40	3	1	7
	FRUITS AND FRUIT PRODUCTS					
215	Apples, raw, me-dium, $2\frac{1}{2}$-inch diameter, about 3 per pound	1 apple	70	Trace	Trace	18
216	Apple brown Betty	1 cup	345	4	8	68
217	Apple juice, bot-tled or canned	1 cup	120	Trace	Trace	30
	Applesauce, canned:					
218	Sweetened	1 cup	230	1	Trace	60
219	Unsweetened or artificially sweetened	1 cup	100	Trace	Trace	26
220	Applesauce and apricots, canned, strained or junior (baby food)	1 ounce	25	Trace	Trace	6
	Apricots:					
221	Raw, about 12 per pound	3 apricots	55	1	Trace	14

Item No.	Food and approximate measure		Food Energy	Protein	Fat (total lipid)	Carbohydrate
	FRUITS AND FRUIT PRODUCTS—Cont'd		*Calories*	*Gm.*	*Gm.*	*Gm.*
	Apricots—continued					
	Canned in heavy sirup:					
222	Halves and sirup	1 cup	220	2	Trace	57
223	Halves (medium) and sirup	4 halves; 2 tablespoons sirup	105	1	Trace	27
	Dried:					
224	Uncooked, 40 halves, small	1 cup	390	8	1	100
225	Cooked, unsweetened, fruit and liquid	1 cup	240	5	1	62
226	Apricot nectar, canned	1 cup	140	1	Trace	36
	Avocados, raw:					
	California varieties, mainly Fuerte:					
227	10-ounce avocado, about $3\frac{1}{3}$ by $4\frac{1}{4}$ inches, peeled, pitted	$\frac{1}{2}$ avocado	185	2	18	6
228	$\frac{1}{2}$-inch cubes	1 cup	260	3	26	9
	Florida varieties:					
229	13-ounce avocado, about 4 by 3 inches, peeled, pitted	$\frac{1}{2}$ avocado	160	2	14	11
230	$\frac{1}{2}$-inch cubes	1 cup	195	2	17	13
231	Bananas, raw, 6 by $1\frac{1}{2}$ inches, about 3 per pound	1 banana	85	1	Trace	23
232	Blackberries, raw	1 cup	85	2	1	19
233	Blueberries, raw	1 cup	85	1	1	21

Item No.	Food and approximate measure		Food Energy	Protein	Fat (total lipid)	Carbohydrate
	FRUITS AND FRUIT PRODUCTS—Cont'd		*Calories*	*Gm.*	*Gm.*	*Gm.*
234	Cantaloups, raw; medium, 5-inch diameter, about $1\frac{2}{3}$ pounds	$\frac{1}{2}$ melon	60	1	Trace	14
	Cherries:					
235	Raw, sweet, with stems	1 cup	80	2	Trace	20
236	Canned, red, sour, pitted, heavy sirup	1 cup	230	2	1	59
237	Cranberry juice cocktail, canned	1 cup	160	Trace	Trace	41
238	Cranberry sauce, sweetened, canned, strained	1 cup	405	Trace	1	104
239	Dates, domestic, natural and dry, pitted, cut	1 cup	490	4	1	130
	Figs:					
240	Raw, small, $1\frac{1}{2}$-inch diameter, about 12 per pound	3 figs	90	1	Trace	23
241	Dried, large, 2 by 1 inch	1 fig	60	1	Trace	15
242	Fruit cocktail, canned in heavy sirup, solids and liquid	1 cup	195	1	1	50
	Grapefruit: Raw, medium, $4\frac{1}{4}$-inch diameter, size 64:					
243	White	$\frac{1}{2}$ grapefruit	55	1	Trace	14
244	Pink or red	$\frac{1}{2}$ grapefruit	60	1	Trace	15
245	Raw sections, white	1 cup	75	1	Trace	20

Item No.	Food and approximate measure		Food Energy	Protein	Fat (total lipid)	Carbohydrate
	FRUITS AND FRUIT PRODUCTS—Cont'd		*Calories*	*Gm.*	*Gm.*	*Gm.*
	Grapefruit—continued					
	Canned, white:					
246	Sirup pack, solids and liquid	1 cup	175	1	Trace	44
247	Water pack, solids and liquid	1 cup	70	·1	Trace	18
	Grapefruit juice:					
248	Fresh	1 cup	95	1	Trace	23
	Canned, white:					
249	Unsweetened	1 cup	100	1	Trace	24
250	Sweetened	1 cup	130	1	Trace	32
	Frozen, concentrate, unsweetened:					
251	Undiluted, can 6 fluid ounces	1 can	300	4	1	72
252	Diluted with 3 parts water, by volume	1 cup	100	1	Trace	24
	Frozen, concentrate, sweetened:					
253	Undiluted, can 6 fluid ounces	1 can	350	3	1	85
254	Diluted with 3 parts water, by volume	1 cup	115	1	Trace	28
	Dehydrated:					
255	Crystals, can, net weight 4 ounces	1 can	430	5	1	103
256	Prepared with water (1 pound yields about 1 gallon)	1 cup	100	1	Trace	24

Item No.	Food and approximate measure		Food Energy	Protein	Fat (total lipid)	Carbohydrate
	FRUITS AND FRUIT PRODUCTS—Cont'd		*Calories*	*Gm.*	*Gm.*	*Gm.*
	Grapes, raw:					
257	American type (slip skin), such as Concord, Delaware, Niagara, Catawba, and Scuppernong	1 cup	65	1	1	15
258	European type (adherent skin), such as Malaga, Muscat, Thompson, Seedless, Emperor, and Flame Tokay	1 cup	95	1	Trace	25
259	Grape juice, bottled or canned	1 cup	165	1	Trace	42
260	Lemons, raw, medium, $2\frac{1}{5}$-inch diameter, size 150	1 lemon	20	1	Trace	6
	Lemon juice:					
261	Fresh	1 cup	60	1	Trace	20
262		1 tablespoon	5	Trace	Trace	1
263	Canned, unsweetened	1 cup	55	1	Trace	19
	Lemonade concentrate, frozen, sweetened:					
264	Undiluted, can, 6 fluid ounces	1 can	430	Trace	Trace	112
265	Diluted with $4\frac{1}{3}$ parts water, by volume	1 cup	110	Trace	Trace	28
	Lime juice:					
266	Fresh	1 cup	65	1	Trace	22
267	Canned	1 cup	65	1	Trace	22
	Limeade concentrate, frozen, sweetened:					
268	Undiluted, can, 6 fluid ounces	1 can	410	Trace	Trace	108

Item No.	Food and approximate measure		Food Energy	Protein	Fat (total lipid)	Carbohydrate
			Calories	Gm.	Gm.	Gm.
	FRUITS AND FRUIT PRODUCTS—Cont'd					
	Limeade concentrate, frozen, sweetened—continued					
269	Diluted with $4\frac{1}{3}$ parts water, by volume	1 cup	105	Trace	Trace	27
	Oranges, raw:					
270	California, navel (winter), $2\frac{4}{5}$-inch diameter, size 88	1 orange	60	2	Trace	16
271	Florida, all varieties, 3-inch diameter	1 orange	75	1	Trace	19
	Orange juice:					
	Fresh:					
272	California, Valencia (summer)	1 cup	115	2	1	26
	Florida varieties:					
273	Early and mid-season	1 cup	100	1	Trace	23
274	Late season, Valencia	1 cup	110	1	Trace	26
275	Canned, unsweetened	1 cup	120	2	Trace	28
	Frozen concentrate:					
276	Undiluted, can, 6 fluid ounces	1 can	330	5	Trace	80
277	Diluted with 3 parts water, by volume	1 cup	110	2	Trace	27
	Dehydrated:					
278	Crystals, can, net weight 4 ounces	1 can	430	6	2	100
279	Prepared with water, 1 pound yields about 1 gallon	1 cup	115	1	Trace	27

Item No.	Food and approximate measure		Food Energy	Protein	Fat (total lipid)	Carbohydrate
	FRUITS AND FRUIT PRODUCTS—Cont'd		Calories	Gm.	Gm.	Gm.
	Orange and grapefruit juice:					
	Frozen concentrate:					
280	Undiluted, can, 6 fluid ounces	1 can	325	4	1	78
281	Diluted with 3 parts water, by volume	1 cup	110	1	Trace	26
282	Papayas, raw, $\frac{1}{2}$-inch cubes	1 cup	70	1	Trace	18
	Peaches:					
	Raw:					
283	Whole, medium, 2-inch diameter, about 4 per pound	1 peach	35	1	Trace	10
284	Sliced	1 cup	65	1	Trace	16
	Canned, yellow-fleshed, solids and liquid:					
	Sirup pack, heavy:					
285	Halves or slices	1 cup	200	1	Trace	52
286	Halves (medium) and sirup	2 halves and 2 tablespoons sirup	90	Trace	Trace	24
287	Water pack	1 cup	75	1	Trace	20
288	Strained or chopped (baby food)	1 ounce	25	Trace	Trace	6
	Dried:					
289	Uncooked	1 cup	420	5	1	109
290	Cooked, unsweetened, 10–12 halves and 6 tablespoons liquid	1 cup	220	3	1	58
	Frozen:					
291	Carton, 12 ounces, not thawed	1 carton	300	1	Trace	77

Item No.	Food and approximate measure		Food Energy	Protein	Fat (total lipid)	Carbohydrate
	FRUITS AND FRUIT PRODUCTS—Cont'd		Calories	Gm.	Gm.	Gm.
	Peaches—continued Frozen:					
292	Can, 16 ounces, not thawed	1 can	400	2	Trace	103
293	Peach nectar, canned	1 cup	120	Trace	Trace	31
	Pears:					
294	Raw, 3 by 2½-inch diameter	1 pear	100	1	1	25
	Canned, solids and liquid: Sirup pack, heavy:					
295	Halves or slices	1 cup	195	1	1	50
296	Halves (medium) and sirup	2 halves and 2 tablespoons sirup	90	Trace	Trace	23
297	Water pack	1 cup	80	Trace	Trace	20
298	Strained or chopped (baby food)	1 ounce	20	Trace	Trace	5
299	Pear nectar, canned	1 cup	130	1	Trace	33
300	Persimmons, Japanese or kaki, raw, seedless, 2½-inch diameter	1 persimmon	75	1	Trace	20
	Pineapple:					
301	Raw, diced	1 cup	75	1	Trace	19
	Canned, heavy sirup pack, solids and liquid:					
302	Crushed	1 cup	195	1	Trace	50
303	Sliced, slices and juice	2 small or 1 large and 2 tablespoons juice	90	Trace	Trace	24
304	Pineapple juice, canned	1 cup	135	1	Trace	34

Item No.	Food and approximate measure		Food Energy	Protein	Fat (total lipid)	Carbohydrate
	FRUITS AND FRUIT PRODUCTS—Cont'd		Calories	Gm.	Gm.	Gm.
	Plums, all except prunes:					
305	Raw, 2-inch diameter, about 2 ounces	1 plum	25	Trace	Trace	7
	Canned, sirup pack (Italian prunes):					
306	Plums (with pits) and juice	1 cup	205	1	Trace	53
307	Plums (without pits) and juice	3 plums and 2 tablespoons juice	100	Trace	Trace	26
	Prunes, dried, "softenized," medium:					
308	Uncooked	4 prunes	70	1	Trace	18
309	Cooked, unsweetened, 17–18 prunes and $\frac{1}{3}$ cup liquid	1 cup	295	2	1	78
310	Prunes with tapioca, canned, strained or junior (baby food)	1 ounce	25	Trace	Trace	6
311	Prune juice, canned	1 cup	200	1	Trace	49
312	Raisins, dried	1 cup	460	4	Trace	124
	Raspberries, red:					
313	Raw	1 cup	70	1	1	17
314	Frozen, 10-ounce carton, not thawed	1 carton	275	2	1	70
315	Rhubarb, cooked, sugar added	1 cup	385	1	Trace	98
	Strawberries:					
316	Raw, capped	1 cup	55	1	1	13

Item No.	Food and approximate measure		Food Energy	Protein	Fat (total lipid)	Carbohydrate
	FRUITS AND FRUIT PRODUCTS—Cont'd		Calories	Gm.	Gm.	Gm.
	Strawberries—continued					
317	Frozen, 10-ounce carton, not thawed	1 carton	310	1	1	79
318	Frozen, 16-ounce can, not thawed	1 can	495	2	1	126
319	Tangerines, raw, medium, 2½-inch diameter, about 4 per pound	1 tangerine	40	1	Trace	10
	Tangerine juice:					
320	Canned, un-sweetened	1 cup	105	1	Trace	25
	Frozen concentrate:					
321	Undiluted, can, 6 fluid ounces	1 can	340	4	1	80
322	Diluted with 3 parts water, by volume	1 cup	115	1	Trace	27
323	Watermelon, raw, wedge, 4 by 8 inches (1/16 of 10 by 16-inch melon, about 2 pounds with rind)	1 wedge	115	2	1	27
	GRAIN PRODUCTS					
324	Barley, pearled, light, uncooked	1 cup	710	17	2	160
325	Biscuits, baking powder with en-riched flour, 2½-inch diameter	1 biscuit	140	3	6	17
326	Bran flakes (40 per-cent bran) added thiamine	1 ounce	85	3	1	23

Item No.	Food and approximate measure		Food Energy	Protein	Fat (total lipid)	Carbohydrate
	GRAIN PRODUCTS—Cont'd		*Calories*	*Gm.*	*Gm.*	*Gm.*
	Breads:					
327	Boston brown bread, slice, 3 by $\frac{3}{4}$ inch	**1 slice**	100	3	**1**	22
	Cracked-wheat bread:					
328	Loaf, 1-pound, 20 slices	**1 loaf**	1,190	39	10	236
329	Slice	**1 slice**	60	2	1	12
	French or Vienna bread:					
330	Enriched, 1-pound loaf	**1 loaf**	1,315	41	14	251
331	Unenriched, 1-pound loaf	**1 loaf**	1,315	41	14	251
	Italian bread:					
332	Enriched, 1-pound loaf	**1 loaf**	1,250	41	4	256
333	Unenriched, 1-pound loaf	**1 loaf**	1,250	41	4	256
	Raisin bread:					
334	Loaf, 1-pound, 20 slices	**1 loaf**	1,190	30	13	243
335	Slice	**1 slice**	60	2	1	12
	Rye bread:					
	American, light ($\frac{1}{3}$ rye, $\frac{2}{3}$ wheat):					
336	Loaf, 1-pound, 20 slices	**1 loaf**	1,100	41	5	236
337	Slice	**1 slice**	55	2	Trace	12
338	Pumpernickel, loaf, 1-pound	**1 loaf**	1,115	41	5	241
	White bread, enriched:					
	1 to 2 percent nonfat dry milk:					
339	Loaf, 1-pound, 20 slices	**1 loaf**	1,225	39	15	229
340	Slice	**1 slice**	60	2	1	12

Item No.	Food and approximate measure		Food Energy	Pro-tein	Fat (total lipid)	Car-bohy-drate
	GRAIN PRODUCTS–Cont'd		*Calo-ries*	*Gm.*	*Gm.*	*Gm.*
	Breads–continued					
	White bread, enriched:					
	3 to 4 percent nonfat dry milk:					
341	Loaf, 1-pound	1 loaf	1,225	39	15	229
342	Slice, 20 per loaf	1 slice	60	2	1	12
343	Slice, toasted	1 slice	60	2	1	12
344	Slice, 26 per loaf	1 slice	45	1	1	9
	5 to 6 percent nonfat dry milk:					
345	Loaf, 1-pound, 20 slices	1 loaf	1,245	41	17	228
346	Slice	1 slice	65	2	1	12
	White bread, unenriched:					
	1 to 2 percent nonfat dry milk:					
347	Loaf, 1-pound, 20 slices	1 loaf	1,225	39	15	229
348	Slice	1 slice	60	2	1	12
	3 to 4 percent nonfat dry milk:					
349	Loaf, 1-pound	1 loaf	1,225	39	15	229
350	Slice, 20 per loaf	1 slice	60	2	1	12
351	Slice, toasted	1 slice	60	2	1	12
352	Slice, 26 per loaf	1 slice	45	1	1	9
	5 to 6 percent nonfat dry milk:					
353	Loaf, 1 pound, 20 slices	1 loaf	1,245	41	17	228
354	Slice	1 slice	65	2	1	12
	Whole-wheat bread, made with 2 percent nonfat dry milk:					
355	Loaf, 1-pound, 20 slices	1 loaf	1,105	48	14	216
356	Slice	1 slice	55	2	1	11
357	Slice, toasted	1 slice	55	2	1	11
358	Breadcrumbs, dry, grated	1 cup	345	11	4	65

Item No.	Food and approximate measure		Food Energy	Protein	Fat (total lipid)	Carbohydrate
	GRAIN PRODUCTS—Cont'd		*Calories*	*Gm.*	*Gm.*	*Gm.*
	Cakes:					
359	Angelfood cake; sector, 2-inch ($\frac{1}{12}$ of 8-inch-diameter cake)	1 sector	110	3	Trace	24
360	Chocolate cake, chocolate icing; sector, 2-inch ($\frac{1}{16}$ of 10-inch-diameter layer cake)	1 sector	445	5	20	67
361	Fruitcake, dark (made with enriched flour); piece, 2 by 2 by $\frac{1}{2}$ inch	1 piece	115	1	5	18
362	Gingerbread (made with enriched flour); piece, 2 by 2 by 2 inches	1 piece	175	2	6	29
	Plain cake and cupcakes, without icing:					
363	Piece, 3 by 2 by $1\frac{1}{2}$ inches	1 piece	200	2	8	31
364	Cupcake, $2\frac{3}{4}$-inch diameter	1 cupcake	145	2	6	22
	Plain cake and cupcakes, with chocolate icing:					
365	Sector, 2-inch ($\frac{1}{16}$ of 10-inch-layer cake)	1 sector	370	4	14	59
366	Cupcake, $2\frac{3}{4}$-inch diameter	1 cupcake	185	2	7	30
367	Poundcake, old-fashioned (equal weights flour, sugar, fat, eggs); slice, $2\frac{3}{4}$ by 3 by $\frac{5}{8}$ inch	1 slice	140	2	9	14

Item No.	Food and approximate measure		Food Energy	Protein	Fat (total lipid)	Carbohydrate
	GRAIN PRODUCTS—Cont'd		*Calories*	*Gm.*	*Gm.*	*Gm.*
	Cakes—continued					
368	Sponge cake; sector, 2-inch ($\frac{1}{12}$ of 8-inch-diameter cake)	1 sector	120	3	2	22
	Cookies:					
369	Plain and assorted, 3-inch diameter	1 cooky	120	1	5	18
370	Fig bars, small	1 fig bar	55	1	1	12
371	Corn, rice and wheat flakes, mixed, added nutrients	1 ounce	110	2	Trace	24
	Corn flakes, added nutrients:					
372	Plain	1 ounce	110	2	Trace	24
373	Sugar-covered	1 ounce	110	1	Trace	26
	Corn grits, degermed, cooked:					
374	Enriched	1 cup	120	3	Trace	27
375	Unenriched	1 cup	120	3	Trace	27
	Cornmeal, white or yellow, dry:					
376	Whole ground, unbolted	1 cup	420	11	5	87
377	Degermed, enriched	1 cup	525	11	2	114
378	Corn muffins, made with enriched degermed cornmeal and enriched flour; muffin, $2\frac{3}{4}$-inch diameter	1 muffin	150	3	5	23
379	Corn, puffed, presweetened, added nutrients	1 ounce	110	1	Trace	26
380	Corn, shredded, added nutrients	1 ounce	110	2	Trace	25
	Crackers:					
381	Graham, plain	4 small or 2 medium	55	1	1	10

Item No.	Food and approximate measure		Food Energy	Protein	Fat (total lipid)	Carbohydrate
	GRAIN PRODUCTS—Cont'd		*Calories*	*Gm.*	*Gm.*	*Gm.*
	Crackers—continued					
382	Saltines, 2 inches square	2 crackers	35	1	1	6
	Soda:					
383	Cracker, 2½-inches square	2 crackers	50	1	1	8
384	Oyster crackers	10 crackers	45	1	1	7
385	Cracker meal	1 tablespoon	45	1	1	7
386	Doughnuts, cake type	1 doughnut	125	1	6	16
387	Farina, regular, enriched, cooked	1 cup	100	3	Trace	21
	Macaroni, cooked:					
	Enriched:					
388	Cooked, firm stage (8 to 10 minutes; undergoes additional cooking in a food mixture)	1 cup	190	6	1	39
389	Cooked until tender	1 cup	155	5	1	32
	Unenriched:					
390	Cooked, firm stage (8 to 10 minutes; undergoes additional cooking in a food mixture)	1 cup	190	6	1	39
391	Cooked until tender	1 cup	155	5	1	32
392	Macaroni (enriched) and cheese, baked	1 cup	470	18	24	44

Item No.	Food and approximate measure		Food Energy	Protein	Fat (total lipid)	Carbohydrate
	GRAIN PRODUCTS—Cont'd		Calories	Gm.	Gm.	Gm.
393	Muffins, with enriched white flour; muffin, 2¾-inch diameter	1 muffin	140	4	5	20
	Noodles (egg noodles), cooked:					
394	Enriched	1 cup	200	7	2	37
395	Unenriched	1 cup	200	7	2	37
396	Oats (with or without corn) puffed, added nutrients	1 ounce	115	3	2	21
397	Oatmeal or rolled oats, regular or quick-cooking, cooked	1 cup	130	5	2	23
	Pancakes (griddlecakes), 4-inch diameter:					
398	Wheat, enriched flour (home recipe)	1 cake	60	2	2	9
399	Buckwheat (buckwheat pancake mix, made with egg and milk)	1 cake	55	2	2	6
	Piecrust, plain baked:					
	Enriched flour:					
400	Lower crust, 9-inch shell	1 crust	675	8	45	59
401	Double crust, 9-inch pie	1 double crust	1,350	16	90	118
	Unenriched flour:					
402	Lower crust, 9-inch shell	1 crust	675	8	45	59
403	Double crust, 9-inch pie	1 double crust	1,350	16	90	118
	Pies (piecrust made with unenriched flour); sector, 4-inch, ⅐ of 9-inch-diameter pie:					
404	Apple	1 sector	345	3	15	51
405	Cherry	1 sector	355	4	15	52

Item No.	Food and approximate measure		Food Energy	Protein	Fat (total lipid)	Carbohydrate
	GRAIN PRODUCTS—Cont'd		*Calories*	*Gm.*	*Gm.*	*Gm.*
	Pies (piecrust made with unenriched flour); sector, 4-inch, $\frac{1}{7}$ of 9-inch-diameter pie—continued					
406	Custard	1 sector	280	8	14	30
407	Lemon meringue	1 sector	305	4	12	45
408	Mince	1 sector	365	3	16	56
409	Pumpkin	1 sector	275	5	15	32
410	Pizza (cheese); $5\frac{1}{2}$-inch sector; $\frac{1}{8}$ of 14-inch-diameter pie	1 sector	185	7	6	27
411	Popcorn, popped, with added oil and salt	1 cup	65	1	3	8
412	Pretzels, small stick	5 sticks	20	Trace	Trace	4
	Rice, white (fully milled or polished), cooked:					
413	Common commercial varieties, all types	1 cup	185	3	Trace	41
414	Long grain, parboiled	1 cup	185	4	Trace	41
415	Rice, puffed, added nutrients (without salt)	1 cup	55	1	Trace	13
416	Rice flakes, added nutrients	1 cup	115	2	Trace	26
	Rolls:					
	Plain, pan; 12 per 16 ounces:					
417	Enriched	1 roll	115	3	2	20
418	Unenriched	1 roll	115	3	2	20
419	Hard, round; 12 per 22 ounces	1 roll	160	5	2	31
420	Sweet, pan; 12 per 18 ounces	1 roll	135	4	4	21
421	Rye wafers, whole grain, $1\frac{7}{8}$ by $3\frac{1}{2}$ inches	2 wafers	45	2	Trace	10

Item No.	Food and approximate measure	Food Energy	Protein	Fat (total lipid)	Carbohydrate
	GRAIN PRODUCTS—Cont'd	Calories	Gm.	Gm.	Gm.
	Spaghetti:				
	Cooked, tender stage (14 to 20 minutes):				
422	Enriched 1 cup	155	5	1	32
423	Unenriched 1 cup	155	5	1	32
424	Spaghetti with 1 cup meat balls in tomato sauce (home recipe)	335	19	12	39
425	Spaghetti in tomato 1 cup sauce with cheese (home recipe)	260	9	9	37
426	Waffles, with enriched flour, $\frac{1}{2}$ by $4\frac{1}{2}$ by $5\frac{1}{2}$ inches 1 waffle	210	7	7	28
	Wheat, puffed:				
427	With added 1 ounce nutrients (without salt)	105	4	Trace	22
428	With added 1 ounce nutrients, with sugar and honey	105	2	1	25
429	Wheat, rolled; 1 cup cooked	175	5	1	40
430	Wheat, shredded, 1 ounce plain (long, round, or bite-size)	100	3	1	23
431	Wheat and malted 1 ounce barley flakes, with added nutrients	110	2	Trace	24
432	Wheat flakes, with 1 ounce added nutrients	100	3	Trace	23
	Wheat flours:				
433	Whole wheat, 1 cup from hard wheats, stirred	400	16	2	85
	All purpose or family flour:				
434	Enriched, sifted 1 cup	400	12	1	84

Item No.	Food and approximate measure		Food Energy	Protein	Fat (total lipid)	Carbohydrate
	GRAIN PRODUCTS—Cont'd		*Calories*	*Gm.*	*Gm.*	*Gm.*
	Wheat flours—continued					
	All purpose or family flour:					
435	Unenriched, sifted	1 cup	400	12	1	84
436	Self-rising, enriched	1 cup	385	10	1	82
437	Cake, or pastry flour, sifted	1 cup	365	8	1	79
438	Wheat germ, crude, commercially milled	1 cup	245	18	7	32
	FATS, OILS					
	Butter, 4 sticks per pound:					
439	Sticks, 2	1 cup	1,625	1	184	1
440	Stick, $\frac{1}{8}$	1 tablespoon	100	Trace	11	Trace
441	Pat or square (64 per pound)	1 pat	50	Trace	6	Trace
	Fats, cooking:					
442	Lard	1 cup	1,985	0	220	0
443		1 tablespoon	125	0	14	0
444	Vegetable fats	1 cup	1,770	0	200	0
445		1 tablespoon	110	0	12	0
	Margarine, 4 sticks per pound:					
446	Sticks, 2	1 cup	1,635	1	184	1
447	Stick, $\frac{1}{8}$	1 tablespoon	100	Trace	11	Trace
448	Pat or square (64 per pound)	1 pat	50	Trace	6	Trace
	Oils, salad or cooking:					
449	Corn	1 tablespoon	125	0	14	0
450	Cottonseed	1 tablespoon	125	0	14	0
451	Olive	1 tablespoon	125	0	14	0
452	Soybean	1 tablespoon	125	0	14	0
	Salad dressings:					
453	Blue cheese	1 tablespoon	80	1	8	1
454	Commercial, mayonnaise type	1 tablespoon	65	Trace	6	2

Item No.	Food and approximate measure		Food Energy	Protein	Fat (total lipid)	Carbohydrate
	FATS, OILS—Cont'd		*Calories*	*Gm.*	*Gm.*	*Gm.*
	Salad dressings—continued					
455	French	1 tablespoon	60	Trace	6	3
456	Home-cooked	1 tablespoon	30	1	2	3
457	Mayonnaise	1 tablespoon	110	Trace	12	Trace
458	Thousand Island	1 tablespoon	75	Trace	8	2
	SUGARS, SWEETS					
	Candy:					
459	Caramels	1 ounce	115	1	3	22
460	Chocolate, milk, plain	1 ounce	150	2	9	16
461	Fudge, plain	1 ounce	115	1	3	21
462	Hard candy	1 ounce	110	0	Trace	28
463	Marshmallows	1 ounce	90	1	Trace	23
464	Chocolate sirup, thin type	1 tablespoon	50	Trace	Trace	13
465	Honey, strained or extracted	1 tablespoon	65	Trace	0	17
466	Jams and preserves	1 tablespoon	55	Trace	Trace	14
467	Jellies	1 tablespoon	55	Trace	Trace	14
	Molasses, cane:					
468	Light (first extraction)	1 tablespoon	50	–	–	13
469	Blackstrap (third extraction)	1 tablespoon	45	–	–	11
470	Sirup, table blends (chiefly corn, light, and dark)	1 tablespoon	60	0	0	15
	Sugars (cane or beet):					
471	Granulated	1 cup	770	0	0	199
472		1 tablespoon	45	0	0	12
473	Lump, $1\frac{1}{8}$ by $\frac{3}{4}$ by $\frac{3}{8}$ inch	1 lump	25	0	0	6
474	Powdered, stirred	1 cup	495	0	0	127
475	before measuring	1 tablespoon	30	0	0	8

Item No.	Food and approximate measure		Food Energy	Protein	Fat (total lipid)	Carbohydrate
	SUGARS, SWEETS—Cont'd		*Calories*	*Gm.*	*Gm.*	*Gm.*
	Sugars (cane or beet)—continued					
476	Brown, firm-	1 cup	820	0	0	212
477	packed	1 tablespoon	50	0	0	13
	MISCELLANEOUS ITEMS					
478	Beer (average 3.6 percent alcohol by weight)	1 cup	100	1	0	9
	Beverages, carbonated:					
479	Cola type	1 cup	95	0	0	24
480	Ginger ale	1 cup	70	0	0	18
481	Bouillon cube, $\frac{5}{8}$ inch	1 cube	5	1	Trace	Trace
	Chili powder. *See* Vegetables, peppers					
482	Chili sauce (mainly tomatoes)	1 tablespoon	20	Trace	Trace	4
	Chocolate:					
483	Bitter or baking	1 ounce	145	3	15	8
484	Sweet	1 ounce	150	1	10	16
	Cider. *See* Fruits, apple juice					
	Gelatin, dry:					
485	Plain	1 tablespoon	35	9	Trace	—
486	Dessert powder 3-ounce package	½ cup	315	8	0	75
	Gelatin dessert, ready-to-eat:					
487	Plain	1 cup	140	4	0	34
488	With fruit	1 cup	160	3	Trace	40
	Olives, pickled:					
489	Green	4 medium or 3 extra large or 2 giant	15	Trace	2	Trace
490	Ripe: Mission	3 small or 2 large	15	Trace	2	Trace

Item No.	Food and approximate measure		Food Energy	Protein	Fat (total lipid)	Carbohydrate
	MISCELLANEOUS ITEMS—Cont'd		*Calories*	*Gm.*	*Gm.*	*Gm.*
	Pickles, cucumber:					
491	Dill, large, 4 by $1\frac{3}{4}$ inches	1 pickle	15	1	Trace	3
492	Sweet, $2\frac{3}{4}$ by $\frac{3}{4}$ inches	1 pickle	30	Trace	Trace	7
	Popcorn. *See* Grain products					
493	Sherbet, orange	1 cup	260	2	2	59
	Soups, canned; ready-to-serve (prepared with equal volume of water):					
494	Bean with pork	1 cup	170	8	6	22
495	Beef noodle	1 cup	70	4	3	7
496	Beef bouillon, broth, consomme	1 cup	30	5	0	3
497	Chicken noodle	1 cup	65	4	2	8
498	Clam chowder	1 cup	85	2	3	13
499	Cream soup (mushroom)	1 cup	135	2	10	10
500	Minestrone	1 cup	105	5	3	14
501	Pea, green	1 cup	130	6	2	23
502	Tomato	1 cup	90	2	2	16
503	Vegetable with beef broth	1 cup	80	3	2	14
504	Starch (cornstarch)	1 cup	465	Trace	Trace	112
505		1 tablespoon	30	Trace	Trace	7
506	Tapioca, quick-cooking granulated, dry, stirred before measuring	1 cup	535	1	Trace	131
507		1 tablespoon	35	Trace	Trace	9
508	Vinegar	1 tablespoon	2	0	–	1
509	White sauce, medium	1 cup	430	10	33	23
	Yeast: Baker's:					
510	Compressed	1 ounce	25	3	Trace	3
511	Dry active	1 ounce	80	10	Trace	11

Item No.	Food and approximate measure	Food Energy	Protein	Fat (total lipid)	Carbohydrate
	MISCELLANEOUS ITEMS—Cont'd	*Calories*	*Gm.*	*Gm.*	*Gm.*
	Yeast—continued				
512	Brewer's, dry, 1 tablespoon debittered	25	3	Trace	3
	Yoghurt. *See* Milk, cream, cheese; related products				

Index